Medical Microbiology

QUALITY COST AND CLINICAL RELEVANCE

QUALITY CONTROL METHODS IN THE CLINICAL LABORATORY

Series Editor: **Byron A. Myhre, M.D., Ph.D.**
Harbor General Hospital (UCLA)
Torrance, California

Medical Microbiology: Quality Cost and Clinical Relevance

Raymond C. Bartlett, M.D.

Medical Microbiology

QUALITY COST AND CLINICAL RELEVANCE

Raymond C. Bartlett, M.D.

Director, Division of Microbiology
Department of Pathology
Hartford Hospital
Hartford, Connecticut

Formerly Chairman, Council on Microbiology,
Commission on Continuing Education,
American Society of Clinical Pathologists

Certificant: Anatomic and Clinical Pathology,
American Board of Pathology

Diplomate: Public Health and Medical Laboratory Microbiology
American Board of Medical Microbiology

A WILEY BIOMEDICAL-HEALTH PUBLICATION

JOHN WILEY & SONS,   **New York • London • Sydney • Toronto**

Library of Congress Cataloging in Publication Data:

Bartlett, Raymond C. 1930–
  Medical microbiology

  (Quality control methods in the clinical
laboratory) (A Wiley biomedical health publication)
  Bibliography: p.
  1. Medical microbiology. 2. Medical
laboratories—Management. I. Title.
[DNLM: 1. Hospital administration. 2. Laboratories.
3. Microbiology. QY23 B291m 1974]

QR46.B36   658′.91′ 61601   73-18482
ISBN 0-471-05475-5

Printed in the United States of America

10 9 8 7 6 5 4 3 2 1

To

The personnel of the author's laboratory without whose
perserverance and creative support the principles set
forth in this book could not have been developed or tested.

Foreword

Clinical diagnostic microbiology is an exceedingly wide field that is being constantly extended both in breadth and in depth. Evaluation as to whether additional diagnostic procedures should be incorporated into the routine schemata employed by the laboratory depends on many factors, but the decisions should be concordant with the goals of the clinical diagnostic microbiology laboratory. The major goal of the clinical diagnostic laboratory is to provide information of maximal clinical or epidemiological usefulness as rapidly as is consistent with acceptable accuracy and minimal cost. In many ways, the maxim attributed to General Nathan B. Forrest over 100 years ago, "get there first with the most . . . ," is directly applicable to the clinical diagnostic microbiology laboratory. This major goal differs from that of the reference laboratory, which attempts to provide the most definitive diagnostic results without particular reference to the time required in the performance of diagnostic procedures. Appreciation of these differences is essential both to the clinician and to the microbiologist.

In preparing this book on *Medical Microbiology,* Dr. Bartlett has brought into clear perspective many of the dilemmas that are faced by both the diagnostic laboratory microbiologist and the clinician who has requested assistance in obtaining information on which to base clinical decisions. As you read this book, you will encounter such phrases as "good bacteriology is clinically relevant bacteriology," "the most laboratory work and hence the greatest cost often is associated with specimens of the least clinical value," and one should not consider "exhaustive microbiology as an end unto itself." Though lifted out of context these phrases may have the ring of trite platitudes, in context the salient points regarding the processing of specimens and the reporting of results, the performance of antimicrobial susceptibility tests, and the use of culture data in infection control activities are defined.

While the entire book will be of most value to individuals whose major efforts are laboratory oriented, for the physician predominantly concerned with the curative and preventive aspects of infectious diseases this microbiology book has much to offer. All of the views expressed are not above controversy; yet they are clearly stated, documented with data, and should be read by all who provide, regulate, or order diagnostic microbiological procedures.

Jay P. Sanford, M.D., F.A.C.P.
Professor of Internal Medicine and
Chief, Infectious Diseases Service
Department of Internal Medicine
University of Texas Southwestern Medical School
Dallas, Texas

Series Preface

Everyone who directs, works in, or owns a clinical laboratory desires accuracy. The purpose of a laboratory is to obtain correct results. Yet errors do occur—usually in an insidious and cumulative manner. A little deviation in technique or a minor error in reagents or equipment can start a chain of circumstances that leads to drastically inaccurate results. Periodic proficiency-testing programs will disclose such inaccuracies, but can neither pinpoint their causes—when, where, and why the chain of errors began—nor suggest a remedy.

Errors can be prevented only by regular programs that test each reagent, procedure, instrument, and intermediate result to determine if they are within the desired limits. This is the essence of *quality control*. If all procedures are correct, the final result must be valid. If they are not correct, quality control tests will locate the deviation, which can then be immediately corrected.

Quality control also improves the morale of the laboratory staff. Since technical deviations are more readily identified and corrected in the laboratory, gross errors are rarely found by the clinical staff and their respect for and confidence in the laboratory is strengthened. This engenders pride in the laboratory staff, leading to a higher morale, which in turn reduces errors.

The chief beneficiary of quality control is the patient. He is not treated or studied further for a suspected disease "diagnosed" by an erroneous laboratory report. Furthermore, he need not pay for supplementary laboratory tests performed to confirm or deny the validity of the suspected test. Nor need he waste time or be subjected to pain while undergoing these supplementary tests.

The clinician also profits from quality control. The results he receives are accurate and allow him to correctly assess the patient's condition. Thus one area of decision-making—estimating the quality of the test—is eliminated.

This series aims to show the reader how to set up quality control in his laboratory and how to act on the information obtained. This will produce more reliable results and aid everyone—laboratory staff, clinician, and patient.

Byron A. Myhre, M.D., Ph.D.
Professor of Pathology
University of California,
Los Angeles

Los Angeles, California
November 1973

Preface

Numerous authoritative texts on medical microbiology are available. Few, however, provide guidance in laboratory administration. Perhaps this is because administration is often viewed apart from the professional or scientific conduct of the medical microbiology laboratory. Those who have borne the burden of administrative decision in this area will affirm the increase in time and effort consumed by this responsibility. Increasing complexity of interaction between laboratory workers, medical staffs, hospital administration, government, and the public will demand greater administrative proficiency of those responsible for operating medical microbiology laboratories.

The principles set forth in this book have been developed and tested in the clinical microbiology laboratory of an institution with an established reputation as one of the nation's largest and most efficient community hospitals dedicated primarily to patient care. Many of the recommendations are empirical; few are supported with published observations. They have been provided to allow concentration of laboratory resources on work which we believe will produce the most benefit for patient care at the lowest cost. Numerous technologists and microbiologists who have found themselves isolated within their institutions, without the authority to impose controls that they believed to be essential, anxiously have sought the kind of guidance which is offered in this book.

Much of the content is not intended to be useful to clinicians and academicians expert in the diagnosis and treatment of infectious diseases. Criticism is anticipated from some who will claim that the guidelines are arbitrary, self imposed and usurp the prerogative of the physician to order and interpret microbiologic examinations. While these critics may aver that more scientific data should be provided to support introduction of controls, we believe that insufficient scientific data are available to support much of the effort which *is* being expended by clinical laboratories because, as we have often heard, "it *might* provide information of clinical value."

Special acknowledgment is extended to Cheryl Rutz, B.A., M.T., A.S.C.P., who had served our laboratory as quality control technologist and technical supervisor. She independently developed much of the organizational structure of our quality control program and successfully delegated responsibility for conducting the program among other laboratory personnel. George Carrington, M.A., Janice Tetreault, M.T. (A.S.C.P.), and Jeanne Frick, B.A., made substantial contributions. John Sherris, M.D., University of Washington, Martin McHenry, M.D., Cleveland Clinic, Jay P. Sanford, M.D., University of Texas, and Richard Quintiliani, M.D., Hartford Hospital, provided helpful suggestions and criticisms. I am especially grateful for the efforts of my secretary, Jane Gudinkas, in the preparation of this manuscript. John Meyer, II, M.D., Pathologist, Day Kimball Hospital, Putnam, Connecticut, prepared the illustration used in Figure 1-1.

Raymond C. Bartlett, M.D.

Hartford, Connecticut
September 1973

Contents

Illustrations

Medical Microbiology

QUALITY COST AND CLINICAL RELEVANCE

## CHAPTER 1

The Role
of the Medical
Microbiologist
in Health Care

Persons of diverse educational background and experience are making significant contributions to the nation's health care through the supervision and direction of diagnostic medical microbiology laboratories. Few organized postdoctoral training programs exist and financial support for these has been subject to a changing economic and political climate. Graduates of clinical pathology residencies in which both the science of microbiology and its application to diagnosis and treatment has been taught in sufficient depth are equally sparse. The public is fortunate to be provided with medical microbiologists, medical technologists, and occasional persons of apparently irrelevant background who have demonstrated professional dedication and responsibility, in the direction of most of the nation's medical microbiology laboratories. The effectiveness of these workers eloquently testifies to the contemporary recognition that effective professional skills can be acquired through a unique series of life-work circumstances that are combined with strong motivation.

The primary responsibility of the *clinical* microbiologist is to provide a diagnostic laboratory service. Although research, development, and education are important elements of his profession they must never be

1

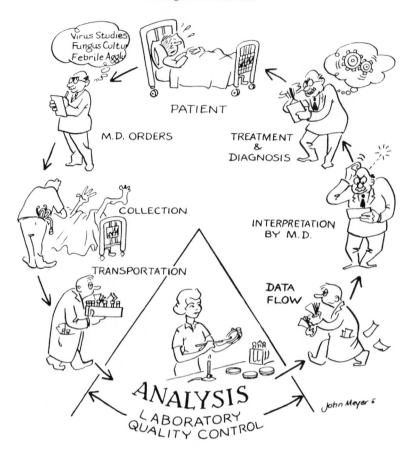

Figure 1-1 Internal laboratory quality control represents only a small portion of the spectrum of activities that affect the quality of patient care. The microbiologist makes many clinically relevant decisions that influence quality performance throughout this spectrum.

allowed to dominate his interest and time. The public health will benefit from the long-range efforts of research microbiologists, but patient care *today* often suffers from the second-class status imposed on diagnostic workers in facilities that are directed and controlled by those whose primary interest is research. Different views are often held and expressed regarding the medical microbiologist's responsibility for the entire spectrum of decisions and actions that affect the way microbiologic information influences the care of the patient. This spectrum is conveniently broken into three categories: (*a*) ordering, collection, and transmission of specimens; (*b*) processing and reporting; and (*c*) interpretation and use of information (Figure 1-1).

Should the nonphysician microbiologist make decisions that involve clinical judgment?

A certain number of physicians in most institutions insist that microbiologists be constrained from such decisions; however, the majority welcome and depend on them. Almost all experienced medical microbiologists believe that they must make certain numbers of decisions involving clinical judgment. The following paragraphs show that all medical microbiologists make decisions that require clinical insight and judgment every day. These decisions are almost always accepted by physicians when they are based on widely acknowledged and clinically substantiated principles. A broader and more authoritative distribution of such guidelines is badly needed. Let us examine the extent to which clinical decisions are already being made in the microbiologist's most proprietary function—processing and reporting.

PROCESSING AND REPORTING

Some microbiologists and physicians have stated that the microbiologist's objective is "to do good bacteriology and leave interpretation up to physicians." What is *good* bacteriology? From a purely technical point of view this could mean complete, definitive, or exhaustive bacteriology. If this is true we cannot afford it. Every medical microbiologist knows that many specimens contain more species of microorganisms than can be enumerated. Even specimens containing pure cultures are reported with some compromise between the clinical demand for a quick response and an academically defensible exclusion of misidentification. Most microbiologists recognize that the number of species found in a clinical specimen is in some way indirectly proportional to the patient care value of the report. A corollary to this is the observation that the most laboratory work and hence the greatest cost, is associated with specimens of the least clinical value. Even worse, *exhaustively good* bacteriology produces irrelevant information, which misleads physicians into erroneous diagnosis and inappropriate therapy. Complete and exhaustive microbiology is also too slow. Often the simple knowledge that a specimen does or does not contain bacteria is the most important clinical consideration (Figure 1-2). As time

	Days					
	1	2	3	4	5	6
Sterile						
Hartford Hospital	86	98	100	100	100	100
Lab X	0	46	64	80	87	100
Growth						
Hartford Hospital	15	87	97	100	100	100
Lab X	0	0	30	56	77	100

Figure 1-2 Comparison of percent of urine specimens reported from the first to the sixth day after being received in the laboratory. Compromise must be reached between exhaustive and clinically useful bacteriology on these specimens. Lab X is a well-known major medical center laboratory.

evolves and the microbiologic report is academically refined, its value in patient care will diminish to the point at which it may be of no importance when documented in the patient's record.

We live in an era of growing government involvement in the evaluation and approval of medical laboratories. In seeking continued "laboratory improvement" there is a great danger of establishing exhaustive microbiology as an end in itself. It is ironic that government, as a representive of the people, may very well bring about significant increases in laboratory costs to the public by insisting on standards for differentiation and identification that are clinically obscure or irrelevant, such as identifiying and reporting *Hemophilus parahemolyticus* from throats; differentiating *Citrobacter* from *Escherichia,* and speciating *Candida* species other than albicans. This trend is discouraging many microbiologists who recognize that the quality of their services will be more effectively improved through careful integration of what is technically feasible with what is clinically important. This is representative of a problem achieving increasing recognition in our society; our technical capabilities are exceeding our ability to apply them effectively and economically to human problems.

Recognition of these facts has forced the medical microbiologist, regardless of background and medical professional status, to make increasing numbers of clinically relevant decisions. He does not perform a third subculture of blood cultures even though certain highly reputable laboratories do and occasional isolates are reported only after this is performed. He does not incubate blood cultures for 3 weeks just because it may be required to isolate *Brucella* or an occasional *Streptococcus viridans* in subacute bacterial endocarditis. He does not perform the morphologic and biochemical tests necessary for the differentiation of normal and mixed flora from body sites commonly contaminated with indigenous bacteria. He does not perform susceptibility tests on all isolates. In deciding what to test he recognizes sites from which certain potential pathogens may be more significant than others. He does not perform routine anaerobic cultures on clinical specimens that are likely to be contaminated with indigenous anaerobic flora or from areas in which anaerobic infection is uncommon. He does not report the presence of small numbers of potential pathogens in the presence of predominating numbers of other potential pathogens from such sites as the respiratory tract although this is often a difficult and arbitrary decision. For most of these decisions the clinical microbiologists may find ample support. If he did not make these decisions microbiology would be too expensive, too slow, and clinically irrelevant.

It has long been recognized, that frequent contact between the microbiologist and the clinician results in a free exchange of information which facilitates both laboratory and clinical decisions. Unfortunately in today's hectic hospital environment many decisions must be made by both the clinician and the microbiologist without such consultation. When the microbiologist is unaware of medically substantial support for his decision he is sometimes tempted to make arbitrary judgments, especially those that would seem clinically *unprovocative*. The presence of multiple species in certain specimens is often obscured in the report to avoid the request that all isolates be speciated and tested for antimicrobial susceptibility. This may lead to the identification and reporting of one, two, or three of many species present when a report of *mixed intestinal* or *cutaneous flora* might be clinically more accurate. Reporting a predominant species in a mixed culture may seem safe, but it is clinically misleading. Often the predominating species is the most rapidly growing organism and may obscure the presence of other significant pathogens. It is in this area that the microbiologist requires substantial medically acknowledged guidelines to support decisions that are clinically relevant and not defensive and misleading. Therefore, *good* bacteriology is *clinically relevant* bacteriology; and clinically relevant bacteriology cannot be performed without making clinically relevant decisions. Can this be extended to the ordering, collection, and transmission of microbiologic specimens?

ORDERING, COLLECTION, AND TRANSMISSION OF SPECIMENS

Many microbiologists feel that their ground is not so firm in this area. Admittedly it is the physician's prerogative to select the time for *collection of the most appropriate material* in relation to the stage of the disease. In spite of this, physicians frequently require guidance. An example is collecting rectal swabs instead of awaiting the report of a stool culture that has been ordered when the patient is unable to produce a specimen. Physicians are dissuaded by the microbiologist from subjecting newborns to venepuncture for serologic tests for syphillis if the mother's serum is nonreactive. They require guidance in the collection of feces, blood, and throat swabs instead of spinal fluid for identifying the agent of viral meningitis. Clinicians often fail to recognize the *effect of contamination* with indigenous flora and must be instructed in proper collection technique by the microbiologist. This is a major problem in the collection of voided urine specimens and sputums. Direct supervision of the collection and transmission of specimens for careful anaerobic culture is a widely recognized essential practice. Other common problems requiring the microbiologist's interaction are the *number of specimens* that should be collected for exclusion of the carrier state of enteric pathogens, the number of blood cultures required in the investigation of a potential case of subacute bacterial endocarditis, or the number of urine or sputum specimens sufficient for excluding a diagnosis of tuberculosis.

The microbiologist also requires the support of acknowledged guidelines, in the defense of requests to perform *tests that he is not prepared to do or for which there is no clinical value.* Centers with experience in isolating *Pneumocystis carinii* have occasionally observed this microorganism in sputum smears. Because of this many clinicians are requesting laboratories that have never observed *Pneumocystis carinii* to perform routine sputum smears for identification of this organism. Microbiologists must indicate the low probability of identification under these circumstances and the need for a needle biopsy of the lung in suspect cases. This problem is representative of a common tendency of physicians to request studies on suboptimal specimens particularly when the disease in question is not the primary suspect. It provides the physician with the specious satisfaction of having covered himself. This is especially true of requests for cultures of fungi and mycobacteria from such inappropriate specimens as feces or highly contaminated material from chronic draining wounds that may be received on swabs. Routine Gram stains on such material as feces or throat swabs are not useful except in selected clinical situations wherein staphylococcal enteritis (clusters of Gram positive cocci), dysentery (monocytes versus neutrophiles), or diphtheria, thrush, and Vincent's infection is suspected. Nevertheless, microbiologists contend that they are required to perform such observations and claim that they lack the acknowledged support to refuse.

Controls must be introduced to promote the delivery of specimens to the laboratory at the most *optimal time for processing.* There is very little justification for performing routine bacteriology on most types of specimens in the hours after midnight. Many microbiologists have established a policy requiring telephone approval before processing such specimens. This eliminates much work that may be performed by less than optimally qualified personnel at these hours. A related problem is the disposition of *duplicate specimens.* This is a growing problem that requires the development of firm policies by microbiologists to control unnecessary duplication of work and needless cost to the patient (see Chapter 4). The microbiologist often utilizes widely acknowledged standards for *delay in transmission* of urine specimens. Unfortunately similar guidelines have not been promulgated for other types of specimens. Unless a transport medium is used, cultures of exudates delayed by more than 4 hours should not be accepted. More than twice the time should not be allowed when a transport medium is used because of changes in the distribution of the bacterial populations present and autolysis of fastidious species.

One of the most difficult situations faced by the microbiologist is the physician's claim that refusal to perform a test on a specimen of poor quality, perhaps improperly collected, or excessively delayed is a disservice to the patient! Physicians often look upon such policies as autocratic and arbitrary rule making by laboratories. However, every physician knows that these standards must be maintained and his reaction is primarily defensive. Microbiologists who have been successful in minimizing confrontations on such matters have established a clear statement of policy which is circulated and verbally reinforced to the medical staff (see Chapter 3).

INTERPRETATION AND UTILIZATION OF MICROBIOLOGIC INFORMATION

Thus it is apparent that the microbiologist makes many clinically relevant decisions in the area of collection and transmission of specimens. What is the extent of his role in the interpretation and utilization of microbiologic information? Does the responsibility of the microbiologist go beyond the use of properly spelled current microbiologic nomenclature in a readable format? Correct nomenclature may mislead physicians. Many microbiologists have elected not to use the term *Streptococcus pneumoniae* to replace *D. pneumoniae* or just plain "pneumococci" because of the certainty of misinterpretation until physicians are familiar with it. The practice of reporting cultures as "contaminated" without speciation is being progressively abandoned. At one time blood cultures containing corynebacteria or *Staphylococcus epidermidis* were construed as being so probably contaminated that they were reported as such. Although the microbiologist cannot make this distinction he can append to a report the *possibility* or *probability* that contamination has occurred if the organism in question is isolated from unusual combinations of media or from limited numbers of the patient's cultures. Disk susceptibility results on *Bacteroides sp.*, *Neisseria sp.*, *Hemophilus sp.*, streptococci, and other species with currently recognized therapeutic regimens are not reported by many microbiologists. This is because of the potential misuse of antibiotics other than those whose consistent effectiveness is recognized as a result of random selection from the susceptibility report. Reporting agents used only for urinary tract infection when tested on isolates from other locations is also dangerous. Although it is not the microbiologist's role to prevent the patient from being treated with an inappropriate antibiotic, this frequently occurs in institutions where proper laboratory policies have not been established. The testing of closely related antimicrobials frequently occurs because of pressure from pharmaceutical representatives and physicians. Fortunately new restricted certification of disks by the Food and Drug Administration will rectify this situation.

It is apparent, therefore, that the microbiologist makes many clinical decisions in the collection, transmission, processing, reporting, and interpretation of clinical microbiological data. Physicians must not look upon these workers as a threat to their clinical prerogative but as a means of improving the ultimate quality of patient care. Greater attention should be given to developing clinically acknowledgeable standards for supporting the decisions of workers in medical microbiology who are faced with a superabundance of academic information and pressure to perform exhaustive, expensive, clinically irrelevant bacteriology, and a general inadequacy of guidelines for a more practical, economical, and clinically meaningful approach.

## CHAPTER 2

Establishing
Clinical Relevance

The preceding chapter emphasized the inseparability of clinical relevance from microbiologic practice in the clinical laboratory. Before beginning a review of methods for standardizing laboratory policies and techniques, let us concentrate on the socioeconomic and clinical considerations toward which laboratory policy should be directed.

The volume of work has increased in the range of 8–10% a year in most hospital microbiology laboratories. There is ample evidence that the volume of work per patient increases proportionately with the academic activity of the institution. A widely acknowledged deficit in American medical education is the increasingly ironic emphasis placed on collecting greater amounts of laboratory data in spite of rising public reaction to health costs and recognition that the cost of laboratory testing has increased at a rate double that of other hospital services. There is little doubt that third parties responsible for reimbursement will look for ways to constrain this seemingly uncontrollable growth. Ceilings have already been placed on laboratory charges in some states.

In Connecticut Blue Cross has replaced its previous "cost plus" reimbursement policy with "prospective reimbursement" which rewards hospitals for reductions in projected costs and penalizes them for exceeding budgets. At this writing Medicare does not permit hospitals to collect more than 7.5% for increases in special service costs from third party payers. A Hospital Cost Commission has been formed in Connecticut. It requires justification for any annual increase in charges above 6%. Cost of living adjustments and higher prices for supplies and services consume most of this. If the medical community continues to demand and obtain annual increases in the volume of laboratory services in the range of 10% per year, regardless of such controls, only increased productivity can prevent a deterioration in the quality of these services. Automation may provide a solution in chemistry and hematology. In microbiology the only alternative to the erosion of quality may be the development of laboratory policies to control excessive and irrelevant utilization.

MONITORING

Much of the increase results from a trend towards microbiologic monitoring of patients who are considered predisposed to infection because of indwelling catheters, endotracheal tubes, tracheostomies, and chronic bronchopulmonary disorders requiring inhalation therapy. Some clinicians believe that the identification of colonizing bacteria on skin or mucous membranes is helpful in the treatment of infections that may occur subsequently. Transition from colonization to infection has been studied (1). A higher incidence of wound infection is associated with colonization of the skin by *Staphylococcus aureus*. Respiratory infection followed by colonization of the respiratory tract by *Klebsiella* (2) or of the skin by *Providencia stuarti* (3) has also been reported. We do not believe that sufficient correlation has been established to verify the value of monitoring colonization as a predictor of the etiology of subsequent infection. Until such evidence is available, clinicians and medical microbiologists should concentrate their resources on detecting agents where and when they cause infection.

OVERUTILIZATION

Several years ago our technologists reported that they were receiving daily urine cultures from a substantial number of patients on one particular service. Investigation revealed that a house officer had written standing orders for daily urine cultures on all patients with indwelling catheters. By the time this circumstance was discovered and corrected one patient's chart contained nearly 100 reports of urine cultures received over a 3-month period. Both doctors and nurses sometimes replicate specimens from patients during the same day because of confusion in carrying out orders. Except for blood and feces, processing more than one specimen per day should be conducted only after consultation between the physician and the microbiologist. In a survey conducted by the author a group of leading hospital laboratories reported that 10% of lower respiratory tract secretion cultures were duplicates.

NEED FOR CONTROLS ON UTILIZATION

Clearly such examples of overutilization dictate the need for controls. Mechanisms for detecting and controlling this problem are described in subsequent chapters. In the section on electronic data processing it is suggested that excess utilization be flagged and reported to the laboratory director for investigation. Hospitals are progressively eliminating the "standing order" that a physician may write with the result that daily medications or laboratory tests continue indefinitely.

Standards should be established, distributed, and enforced to control delay in transmission, improper submission, duplication, and excessive and clinically irrelevant utilization. Later chapters describe methods for accomplishing this. It is often said that the laboratory is doing a disservice to the patient by refusing such specimens. In reality the disservice is being performed by the physician or nurse who submits this kind of material and by the laboratory that accepts and thereby promotes this practice while simultaneously diverting its resources from the evaluation of optimal specimens.

When nonspecific or unusual requests are received with specimens the microbiologist should discuss the matter with the submitting physician. No matter how well priorities are directed toward patient care, time may not permit such personal communication. A promptly rendered report requesting a consultation may be a more efficient means of accomplishing this. In most instances insufficient need or clinical justification exists and physicians ignore the request. In other instances where obscure or ill-defined procedures have been called for by house staff, our petition for consultation directed to the attending physician has evoked the response that he could not justify the request of the house officer.

It is necessary to refrigerate specimens while awaiting either a consultation or a collection of new specimens asked for by the laboratory because of poor quality or improper submission. Some clinicians, pathologists, and microbiologists have not felt that this could be justified because of potential deterioration. We believe that a poorer service is rendered at a greater cost to the patient if laboratory resources are expended in an arbitrary manner on nonspecific requests and specimens of doubtful value.

Performance of microbiologic procedures during the evening or night must be controlled. Some laboratory directors have acquiesced to repeated demands by physicians for moderately comprehensive 24-hour laboratory service. We believe that this is not economically justifiable. Providing these services at night is always more costly. Many tests requested at these hours make no essential contribution to diagnosis and treatment and, therefore, could be performed during regular hours. Too often tests are demanded either because of the physician's insecurity in establishing a diagnosis or for academic curiosity. Discussion of the problem with an informed and sympathetic representative of the laboratory, preferably also a physician, often convinces an otherwise demanding clinician that the results of the test will not significantly affect his management of the patient for the next 6 or 8 hours. Planting a urine culture from a patient who develops signs and symptoms of an acute urinary infection, for which it is desirable to immediately institute therapy, is justifiable at any hour. A simple system should be established to approve processing this type of specimen but simultaneously prevent the submission and inoculation of vast numbers of urine specimens, obtained for routine diagnostic purposes, which happen to land in the laboratory late at night. Procedures that result in the collection of specimens for culture are often performed late in the evening because house officers have been busy with rounds and conferences during regular working hours. One hears and reads a good deal about the value of efficient laboratory testing for shortening and reducing the cost of hospitalization. Preadmission cultures may permit earlier and more specific treatment of infections. We know of no evidence that processing unselected specimens during the night shortens hospitalization.

Quality of service and productivity may also be improved by more selective and clinically relevant application of resources in the microbiology laboratory. If three or four intestinal species are isolated and reported with results of susceptibility testing this information may be of a lesser quality than a report of "mixed intestinal flora." The former report implies to the physician that no other intestinal species exist in the infection (almost certainly not true) and encourages the use of either a combination of antimicrobials or toxic broad spectrum antimicrobials, a conclusion that could have been reached by the latter report, which is quicker and much less expensive for the laboratory to produce.

There is a danger that productivity and quality will be decreased if clinical microbiology is treated as a definitive science. There is general agreement that all who are engaged in the delivery of health care must find ways to make more selective use of resources. The microbiologist who expends laboratory effort to report microbiologic information of an obscure or low order of clinical significance is just as guilty of abusing these resources as the physician who orders vast numbers of laboratory tests and prolongs a patient's hospitalization to rule out improbable diagnoses.

Significant misconceptions and confusion exist about the reporting and interpretation of bacteriologic data from a number of body sites. The following observations are made in the hope that clinicians and those responsible for evaluating laboratory performance will support microbiologists who are discriminating in the use of laboratory resources to provide high quality information at the lowest possible cost.

ANTIMICROBIAL SUSCEPTIBILITY TESTING

A substantial amount of the antimicrobial susceptibility testing that is performed in clinical laboratories is unnecessary and simultaneously generates clinically irrelevant and potentially misleading information. A request for susceptibility testing should be construed as approval for testing if an agent is isolated for which such testing is indicated. It should not cause laboratory workers to arbitrarily test isolates when results are not clinically useful. It would be more helpful if physicians could indicate when susceptibility testing is *not* required but it is doubtful that this would occur often enough to be worth promoting as a means of reducing unnecessary work. In a series of annual national conferences conducted on this subject the panel, of both clinicians and laboratory scientists has never failed to agree unanimously that the decision to perform an antimicrobial susceptibility test belongs in the laboratory. Physicians often object to patients' being billed for susceptibility testing that they did not order. This is no worse than billing the patient for susceptibility testing that is ordered but would not have been performed if the laboratory had the prerogative! We make no extra charge for susceptibility testing. Very few laboratories charge for the additional biochemical tests or serologic work that may be required for identification of a *Salmonella*. Why charge extra for susceptibility tests? Although deletion of this charge may seem acceptable to many laboratory directors and hospital administrators, it requires a compensatory increase in charges for all cultures.

In our laboratory the susceptibility test is not performed routinely on *Neisseria sp., Hemophilus influenzae, Clostridium sp., Streptococcus pneumoniae* (pneumococcus), Group A beta hemolytic streptococci, and indigenous bacteria isolated from the mouth, gastrointestinal (G.I.) tract, vagina, and skin. The cumulative reporting system used in our laboratory (see Chapter 4) allows the recognition of species repeatedly isolated from the same site on sequential days. Susceptibility testing is not repeated until 3 days have elapsed. Twelve of 27 laboratories surveyed by the author conducted susceptibility tests when specimens were received on consecutive days. The other 15 repeated this test after a lapse of 3–7 days. Susceptibility testing is performed on up to three isolates. When more than three isolates are found in equal numbers, cultures are usually reported as mixed without speciation or susceptibility testing (see Wounds, p. 19).

ANAEROBIC CULTURES

Clinicians and microbiologists are becoming increasingly concerned with anaerobic infection. Techniques for isolating and identifying fastidious anaerobes have advanced more rapidly than the development of clinical criteria for rational use of the information that is produced. Although anaerobic infection is an important problem which requires careful clinical and laboratory investigation, most specimens that are collected contain substantial amounts of indigenous oropharyngeal, or cutaneous or intestinal flora, much of which is anaerobic. Routine application of sensitive anaerobic techniques to such specimens often yields a potpourri of aerobic and anaerobic bacteria. Differentiation speciation and reporting of these bacteria have placed a substantially increased demand on laboratory resources. Unless direct anaerobic bacteriology is applied selectively to specimens that have been collected by techniques that specifically exclude contaminating indigenous anaerobic bacteria, laboratories will incur a new wave of increasing cost. More specific additional remarks concerning anaerobic cultures of sputum, urine, and wounds can be found in the sections that follow.

MYCOLOGY

Many specimens are collected on swabs and submitted with the nonspecific request "fungus culture." Applying mycologic techniques to such specimens capable of demonstrating all pathogenic fungi in direct examination and culture is an inappropriate way to expend laboratory resources. Unless proper material is submitted with one or more specific fungi listed on the request slip, we freeze these specimens and stamp the report with a request for consultation.

This policy is well supported by the recognition that suitable methods of direct examination may range from Wright and Giemsa's stain to Methamine silver, Periodic acid Schiff, and KOH preparations, and Gram stain, depending on the agent suspected. Furthermore, incorporating antibiotics and other inhibitory substances in the culture medium significantly affects the isolation of certain fungi and actinomycetes; the importance of their use is dictated by the probability of bacterial contamination. Most physicians do not realize that swabs are inappropriate for fungal culture. Swab collected specimens should always be replaced by more appropriately collected material, with the exception of vaginal cultures for *Candida*.

More than half the time we receive no response to requests for consultation and the specimens are discarded after 72 hours. Follow-up inquiry has revealed that most requests for "fungus culture" result from considering fungal infection as a diagnosis that is improbable but requires exclusion. Often by the time the consultation request is received, interest in the possibility of fungal infection is insufficient to cause the physician to pursue the matter. When physicians call we review the type of specimen that was received and the need for collection of additional material to provide maximum sensitivity for isolation of whichever fungi are suspected. If histoplasma is suspected fresh specimens must be collected because freezing is harmful to this agent. A Gram stain of sputum often reveals that the specimen consists primarily of oropharyngeal material, whereupon the physician is asked to collect more material avoiding oropharyngeal contamination. We request another consultation after three consecutive specimens have been received and processed.

Opportunistic fungi, especially *Candida*, are frequently isolated from routine cultures of respiratory secretions, vagina, and superficial wounds. In all but a few cases this represents insignificant colonization. In the absence of any request for isolation of fungi from these specimens we have established a policy of refrigerating plates for 72 hours and reporting "Yeast isolated, consultation requested for speciation" unless the agent is isolated in pure culture. This eliminates unnecessary effort for speciation in the majority of instances.

MYCOBACTERIA

Smears for mycobacteria may be performed on urine or gastric contents but clinicians must be cognizant of the occurrence of indigenous mycobacteria in these sites. Spinal fluid may be stained for acid-fast bacilli, not by performing a Ziehl-Nielsen on a simple smear but only after building up multiple layers of fluid and allowing sufficient time for drying before applying each loopful. This should be done only after a consultation during which the clinician is informed that smears are rarely positive except in advanced cases and require a tedious staining procedure that necessitates several hours of effort by an experienced worker. In our laboratory a consultation is requested prior to processing more than three consecutive specimens from any site.

Tissue that is received either from surgical biopsies or autopsies frequently is inadequate in amount, contaminated, or fixed in formalin. Swab cultures are entirely inadequate for isolation of fungi or mycobacteria from such specimens. There is a tendency among surgeons to drop lymph nodes into formalin without considering the need for submitting fresh tissue to the microbiology laboratory. Only by refusing swab cultures or requests for isolation of mycobacteria from formalin fixed tissues have we succeeded in establishing a practice of routine submission of a portion of fresh tissue when mycobacterial infection is suspected.

AUTOPSY CULTURES

There are abundant reviews of autopsy microbiology which indicate that proper techniques substantially reduce contamination (4). We require that tissue, not swabs, be submitted from all autopsy tissues. This is first washed repeatedly in sterile saline to eliminate superficially contaminating bacteria and is then ground. If heavy superficial contamination is suspected, the tissue may be washed with alcohol prior to rinsing in saline. It is discouraging to observe a technologist who has spent several days with stacks of plates and racks of tubes attempting to speciate mixed intestinal flora that was introduced into a specimen at the autopsy table. Mixed cultures from autopsies should be reported as such with indication that further work will be performed after consultation from the pathologist or resident responsible for the case. Quantitative culture may be helpful because significant isolates usually exceed 10^4 per milliliter of tissue.

VIROLOGY

Virology represents an area in which maintaining clinical relevance is a new and serious problem. Whether virology is performed by the hospital laboratory or material is submitted to a reference laboratory, controls must be exercised to prevent the submission and processing of specimens labeled only as "Virus studies." A clinical data sheet should be required to provide the virologist with some index of the type of disease suspected. Acute sera should not be titered until a second paired specimen is obtained. In many cases this specimen may never be received because the diagnosis becomes resolved after the collection of the acute serum. The submission of a second specimen within 5 days is usually accidental and could not provide significant changes in titer. This often results from duplication in ordering and is reported out of our laboratory as "See results of specimen submitted on. . . ." The State Health Department and the Center for Disease Control (CDC), which perform many serologic tests not conducted in hospital laboratories, require clinical information that helps to guide them toward the suspected disease and eliminates idle requests.

WOUNDS

Wound cultures derived from lesions that are contaminated with intestinal, cutaneous, or oropharyngeal flora burden the laboratory with unnecessary effort, produce reports that imply infection where there is none, and promote antimicrobial therapy of noninvasive bacteria. The microbiologist finds himself in the dilemma of attempting to isolate and speciate everything that is present, reporting one or two predominating species, or applying his knowledge of relative pathogenicity and concentrating his efforts on the most probable pathogens. Some microbiologists and physicians feel that everything should be reported and that only the clinician can determine which isolates are clinically significant. This is economically unfeasible. Misleading information, which may be misinterpreted, is often reported as a result of this procedure.

Proper collection, labeling, and transport of specimens contributes much to the quality of the microbiologist's report. This can be reviewed with the medical and the nursing staff through conferences and written standards that are conveniently available on all nursing units (see Chapter 3). Despite these efforts we have found that sufficient attention is still not given to the proper cleansing of heavily colonized or contaminated sites.

Labeling was improved after the addition of an extra box on the requisition slip entitled "body site." Nurses may be called on to provide this information if the number is small enough to be handled conveniently. We have found that a tube of Stuarts transport medium is a simple means of keeping swabs moist and protecting anaerobes during transit. Delays of 4–6 hours between collection and delivery to the laboratory are undesirable but are probably not worth austere control efforts. We plant specimens from wounds collected during the night if the technician is called. When no call is made and a specimen is found 6 or more hours later in the morning, we refrigerate it and stamp the report "received after prolonged delay; please submit another specimen." Physicians call in most such instances because specimens have been collected during surgery and cannot be repeated. This policy results in a few additional hours of delay but has a salutary effect on promoting the practice of calling the laboratory for prompt planting during night hours. Physicians and nurses should be periodically instructed on the effects of delay on wound cultures in transport medium. Anaerobes are not optimally protected and multiply slowly while the presence of body fluids and exudate may markedly stimulate growth of coliforms and Proteus species. This distorts the ratio in both the Gram stain and the culture of such specimens and may produce significantly misleading reports. The same is true of mixtures of enteric bacteria, streptococci, and staphylococci. The use of thioglycollate broth or any other nutrient medium for transport of specimens for culture should be condemned because of the marked distortion that occurs in the relative populations of slowly and rapidly growing bacteria prior to inoculation onto plating media.

Routine anaerobic plate culture of all wounds substantially increases the cost of processing these cultures and the information produced is of doubtful clinical value in most cases. The cost of direct anaerobic culture is at least double the charge for processing specimens to which it is applied. Most laboratories could not incubate the large number of anaerobic jars required nor could they apply the amount of time required for identification of the multiple anaerobes that would be isolated from the majority of specimens without additional incubator capacity and personnel. Roll tubes need less space but their handling requires more time and elaborate equipment than the more convenient anaerobic plate technique. Roll tube methods reach lower eH levels than anaerobic jar procedures and increase the isolation of many unfamiliar anaerobic species that are almost always in mixed culture with anaerobic species of established pathogenicity. Until the clinical significance of these unfamiliar species is fully established by research programs, their isolation should not be viewed as justification for the increased cost of this procedure in the majority of microbiology laboratories.

Direct anaerobic culture may be applied to specimens from abdominal wounds or abscesses in any location. It should be applied to collections from body cavities and visceral abscesses. Personnel should be instructed to recognize specimens labeled from sources that might warrant direct anaerobic culture. When in doubt, an experienced laboratory worker or the pathologist may assist in making this decision. Foul smelling material is a clue to the presence of anaerobes. Clinicians must be repeatedly reminded to request an anaerobic culture when anaerobic infection is suspected.

The Gram stain can give rapid information on the quality of material that has been submitted, the presence of a pyogenic exudate, and the type of bacteria present. Yet few physicians order Gram stains or express interest in their content. Although most workers prepare smears from wound specimens, these are usually not stained and examined unless this has been requested. The terse objective reporting of "Gram positive cocci 1+; Gram negative rods 2+, etc." must be interpreted to be of clinical value. Many physicians prefer to await the speciation and susceptibility results of the final culture report because it provides specific instructions for treatment not furnished by the Gram stain report. Several workers have developed reporting systems that correlate Gram stain results with antimicrobial susceptibility profiles and suggest antimicrobials appropriate for the agents observed. Some clinicians have complained that this represents unwarranted meddling by the laboratory in decisions that they are more capable of making independently. This may be true of those who have a large experience in managing infectious diseases but we know of many clinicians who would welcome this information. On innumerable occasions we have examined Gram stains and assisted clinicians in selecting the most appropriate antimicrobial by correlating possible species present with current antimicrobial profiles. In the absence of such a consultation, it is doubtful that strictly objective routine reporting of all Gram stains produces information that most clinicians would use. An alternative would be a slightly expanded description in a more narrative form by an experienced microbiologist. Report slips containing sufficient space or computer reporting programs capable of handling free language entry may permit this to be done when requested by physicians in place of the usual brief morphologic report, or as a part of an expanded report when mixed cultures are observed.

Some laboratories are able to find the time for personnel to correlate all culture results with Gram stains of the direct smear. Many discrepancies are found. This may lead to written or verbal reports of the presence of agents inferred from the Gram stains but not from cultures. One common example is the discovery of Gram negative rods morphologically suggestive of *Bacteroides* and cocci suggestive of *Peptostreptococcus* from specimens on which anaerobic culture was not requested or performed and which produce a few colonies of enteric bacteria on aerobic culture. Thioglycollate or chopped meat broth is likely to be so overgrown with enteric bacteria that anaerobes will not be recovered on subculture. To be practical, examining Gram stains must usually be confined to complicated specimens that contain multiple isolates, or to instances in which physicians request Gram stain results or inquire about the interpretation of reports. In our laboratory, a unique exception is the routine examination of Gram stains of direct smears on all specimens producing sterile cultures. We have repeatedly observed bacteria in cases where a sterile culture by itself would have been quite misleading.

Only about 10% of wound specimens yield sterile cultures in our laboratory. The majority contain two or three isolates; about 15% contain more than three. With the exception of *Streptococcus pyogenes,* aerobic organisms are not reported from broth culture unless the plates are sterile. Anaerobes isolated from broth or anaerobic plate cultures are report along with aerobes isolated from aerobic plates.

For a number of years it has been the policy in our laboratory to report and perform antimicrobial susceptibility tests on up to three isolates from wound cultures. When greater numbers are observed cultures are discussed on daily laboratory rounds with the author. Evaluation begins with inspection of the Gram stain. Frequently there is an abundance of squamous cells and bacteria with no neutrophils. Such specimens have been reported as "Mixed intestinal (or depending on the flora observed: mixed cutaneous; mixed oropharyngeal) flora isolated; Gram stain suggests that material is superficial and that isolates may not be related to infection." When neutrophils are observed an attempt is made to speciate only those isolates that are represented in the Gram stain. If the total number of species observed both in Gram stain and culture exceeds three, the physician is called. Invariably we have been able to convince physicians that complete speciation and antimicrobial susceptibility testing under these circumstances is not worthwhile and that repeat collection with elimination of contaminating and colonizing flora is more likely to produce specific information for guidance of therapy.

Presently we are experimenting with a system for evaluation of specimens from wounds by examination of the Gram stain on the day specimens are received. This is patterned after the system which for several years has been successfully applied to evaluation of specimens of lower respiratory secretions in our laboratory (see Lower Respiratory Secretions, p. 27). A "score" that reflects the relative numbers of neutrophils and squamous cells is used to guide the technologist in processing specimens. Specimens that show squamous cells and no neutrophils achieve a score of "0" and are refrigerated in transport medium for 72 hours. A report is rendered stating: "Superficial material, no evidence of inflammation. Please consult regarding further examination." We believe this expedites collection of better specimens, and reduces unnecessary microbiologic effort productive of useless clinical information. These benefits should outweigh the disadvantage of delaying processing of occasional specimens that may appear to be superficial and without evidence of inflammation but for some unforeseen clinical reason may be justifiably processed.

Specimens that show varying numbers of squamous cells and neutrophils achieve scores of 1 to 3. Gram stains of these specimens are examined for bacteria. Instead of reporting "Gram negative rods 1+" and so on, a more interpretive report is rendered stating: "Preliminary report-Cells, and Bacteria, suggested by Gram stain: Squam. ( ), Neut. ( ), Lymph. ( ), R.B.C. ( ), Strep. ( ), Staph. ( ), Clostrid. ( ), Enteric. ( ), Pseudo. ( ), Neisseria ( ), Bacteroides, Pasteurella, Hemoph. ( )." These specimens are planted. When *Clostridium* or *Bacteroides* are suspected plates are inoculated for direct anaerobic culture. The score guides the technologist in working up isolates from these specimens. Whenever the score is exceeded by the number of isolates, the specimen is discussed on daily laboratory rounds with the author. Invariably these specimens have been reported as "Mixed flora isolated [cutaneous ( ); intestinal ( ); vaginal ( )]. Correlation with Gram stain suggests that these isolates may not relate to infection. Please repeat minimizing superficial flora or consult regarding further examination."

This system has eliminated planting of about 10% of specimens and speciation and antimicrobial sensitivity testing of multiple isolates in an additional 20%. This reduction by one-third in the number of specimens requiring time-consuming bacteriologic effort has provided the time necessary for evaluation of Gram stains of the specimens. The net effect has not been so much to reduce total work but to shift application of effort to work productive of more useful clinical information. Preliminary reporting of species suggested by Gram stain and selective anaerobic culture of specimens showing presumptive anaerobic species are but two examples of the benefits derived from this selective approach.

Alternative practices of reporting one, two, or three predominating isolates from a specimen that contains additional isolates in lesser numbers is misleading because it implies to the physician that other species are not present. It is quite doubtful that specific therapy of an isolate predominating in a mixture of intestinal flora will be more successful than empirical therapy directed at intestinal bacterial flora in general. The reporting of multiple species invariably rules out specific therapy and suggests the use of the same broad spectrum antimicrobials that are likely to be selected on the basis of a report of "mixed intestinal flora." Most physicians recognize that mixed infections generally respond better to debridement and drainage than to broad spectrum antimicrobial therapy. Those who do not are just as likely to use these drugs whether multiple species or "mixed flora" are reported.

BLOOD CULTURE

Blood culture represents the most expensive routine procedure conducted in bacteriology laboratories. There is a wide difference of opinion about the most appropriate procedure and choice of materials. Although many exciting alternatives to conventional blood culture technique have recently appeared, these have been introduced in only a few laboratories and their application to routine diagnostic work has yet to be proved (5).

In a survey of 21 nationally recognized microbiology laboratories the author found that most were experiencing between 5 and 10 culture collections per year per bed (6). Those exceeding 15 were major teaching institutions and those with less than 5 were community hospitals with little or no teaching commitments. A wide range was also observed in the number of blood cultures that could be processed per full-time worker. Although the mean of the laboratories surveyed appeared to fall between 4000 and 8000 collections per worker per year, almost half of the laboratories processed less than this number. This correlated with the number of subcultures performed. The lowest volume of 2000 cultures per worker was reported by the only laboratory that routinely performed four subcultures on all collections. Conversely a laboratory that was able to handle 15,000 collections per worker per year did not perform subcultures routinely. The complexity and resulting cost of processing these specimens is compounded by frequent instances in which inexperienced house staff have collected literally dozens of specimens in a single day. Although the laboratory can establish limitations on the number of blood cultures that it will collect, it is powerless to control the appearance of boxes filled with inoculated blood cultures ready for incubation.

Most of the microbiologists responding to the author's survey reported that they had no control over the number of blood cultures requested by physicians. Furthermore the majority did not feel that it was within their purview to make recommendations on this matter. It is clear that cooperation between microbiologists and physicians with special interest in infectious disease is required to establish acceptable recommendations in many institutions. Most microbiologists believe that three blood cultures per day collected at random intervals or in association with chills and fever is sufficient for the diagnosis of bacteremia. In a study of 206 cases of bacterial endocarditis reported by Werner, 97% of the blood cultures were positive if no previous antibiotics had been given (7). In the presence of previous antimicrobial therapy the yield was reduced to 91%. No patient re-

Collections per Septicemia	Septicemias	Cultures Positive per Septicemia				
		1	2	3	4	5
1	22	22				
2	16	3	13			
3	13	4	3	6		
4	6	0	1	1	4	
5	1	0	1	0	0	0
6	1	0	0	1	0	0
>6	0	0	0	0	0	0
Total	59					

Figure 2-1   In 45 of 59 septicemias in which at least one blood culture was collected, all cultures were positive. The study eliminated clinically apparent septicemia in which no cultures were positive because it could not be established that bacteremia had occurred. In no instance were more than four culture collections required to obtain at least one positive. The statistical probability of obtaining at least one positive culture if the number of collections had been limited was: 28.2/37 (76%) for one collection, 30.3/37 (82%) for two collections, 20.6/21 (98%) for three collections, and 8/8 (100%) for four collections.

quired more than three blood cultures to establish a diagnosis of the etiologic agent of bacterial endocarditis when antimicrobial therapy had not been given previously. When there had been a history of antimicrobial therapy within 2 weeks, no more than seven blood cultures were required.

A study was conducted in the author's laboratory to determine the number of blood cultures required to isolate the etiologic agents in other types of bacteremias (Figure 2-1). In a study of 59 culture positive septicemias none was found in which more than four blood cultures would have been required to demonstrate the infecting organism.

It is generally acknowledged that the bacteremia of bacterial endocarditis is a continuous phenomenon. Although the collection of 40 cc of blood might provide a sufficient sample to isolate the etiologic agent, this is usually divided among several separate collections to minimize the risk of contamination. There is no evidence that any particular interval between collections is optimal. Other than gathering specimens when bacterial showers produce chills and fever, collections at hourly intervals are probably satisfactory. Laboratory workers should not permit themselves to be forced into collecting blood cultures at 5 and 10 minute intervals as is often specified by inexperienced house officers. This usually occurs in instances of acute infection when instituting rapid antimicrobial therapy is of interest. There is no reason to believe that 1 or 2 hours of delay in therapy will affect the outcome in subacute bacterial endocarditis. In acute endocarditis or other acute septicemic conditions rapid initiation of therapy is important. Here one may collect four cultures from two separate venipunctures following which therapy may be instituted immediately.

In conclusion it would appear reasonable to establish four blood cultures per day as the maximum required for a diagnosis of bacteremia in the absence of previous antimicrobial therapy. Collections need not be made at less than hourly intervals except in cases of acute infection where several blood cultures can be collected simultaneously. Patients who have received previous courses of antimicrobial therapy within 2 weeks may require double this number of cultures to establish a diagnosis.

Adequate skin decontamination is required to reduce the number of spurious isolates that are recovered. Using a double skin preparation beginning with an organic iodide solution followed by alcohol is more effective than using either alone.

Although a wide variety of culture media are used, adding sodium polyanethol sulfonate is widely acclaimed. There are as many microbiologists who use penicillinase in blood cultures as there are those who do not. Contamination and deterioration of penicillinase solutions may occur and these materials should be subject to frequent surveillance. It is desirable to maintain at least a 1:10 dilution ratio because of the natural inhibitory titer of serum against most Gram negative bacteria. This also dilutes out the effects of antibiotics.

During the last few years there has been a trend toward reducing the incubation time for blood cultures. The majority of microbiologists continue to incubate for 14 days. The author's laboratory adheres to the more conservative position since clinically significant isolates have occasionally been recovered after 1 week of incubation. In a series of 500 positive blood cultures 12% became positive after 7 days. Five of this percentile were considered clinically significant and seven were contaminants.

It is debatable whether more than two subcultures should be performed during the course of incubation. However, it is certain that failure to routinely subculture results in overlooking important organisms such as *Neisseria gonorrhoeae, Hemophilus influenzae*, or *Streptococcus pneumoniae*. Five of the 21 laboratories surveyed by the author performed three subcultures routinely, and one conducted four. Although it was impossible to establish any typical expression of laboratory practice on this matter, it was concluded that a subculture at 24 hours and again at 7 days is a justifiable minimal standard. There is no doubt that both aerobic and anaerobic cultures should be performed on blood. Only one of the laboratories in the survey did not make this a routine procedure.

It is difficult to determine the actual frequency of contamination in blood cultures. Laboratories have reported anything from 1 to 25%. The isolation of *Corynebacterium sp. Propionibacterium sp., Staphylococcus epidermidis*, and *Bacillus sp.* is usually construed as evidence of cutaneous contamination. It is important to recognize that patients who possess metal or plastic in body cavities or blood vessels, especially in association with neuro- or cardiovascular surgery, are susceptible to infection from these organisms.

Mixed blood cultures that are clinically significant may be more frequent than is generally acknowledged. Although some microbiologists believe that less than 1% of blood cultures are mixed, published data suggest that the frequency may be as high as 24% (8). Six (10%) of the series of 59 septicemias previously referred to from the author's study represented mixed infection. We have observed a patient with bacterial endocarditis from which two strains of *Enterococcus* were isolated, each demonstrating significantly different levels of antimicrobial susceptibility.

There are differences of opinion among microbiologists about reporting blood cultures that appear to be contaminated. Although some accept the term "possible" and/or "probable contamination," many prefer to report the species isolated without any implication of contamination. It is certain that a previous practice of reporting blood cultures containing such organisms as "sterile" should be abandoned because of the increasing recognition of clinically significant infection with these agents. On the other hand omission of any appellation suggesting contamination may result in unnecessary antimicrobial therapy. It may be best to compromise and qualify reports in which the isolation of suspected contaminants occurs in only one of two or more blood cultures as "possibly" or "probably contaminated."

LOWER RESPIRATORY SECRETIONS

A culture of lower respiratory secretions may result in more unnecessary microbiologic effort than any other type of specimen. Recent reports have emphasized a high frequency of colonization of the oropharynx with *Staphylococcus aureus* and Gram negative rods (9). It is well known that the pathogenesis of most cases of pneumonia involve the introduction of bacterial flora from the upper respiratory tract and pharynx into the lower respiratory tract. Collecting sputum that has passed through this region is an illogical means of establishing a bacteriologic diagnosis of pneumonia. It is little more than convenience for the physician and comfort for the patient that sustains the practice. Increasing emphasis is being placed on methods for eliminating the confusion that results from isolation of colonizing oropharyngeal bacteria. These include: washing the sputum, homogenization, tracheal aspiration, tracheal puncture, bronchoscopy, needle aspiration of the lung, and lung biopsy. Some physicians have suggested that sputum specimens should not be collected from patients who have been hospitalized for more than 2 days because of the high frequency of pharyngeal colonization with potential pulmonary pathogens. Recent publications have commented on the limitations of diagnosing pneumococcal pneumonia by demonstrating the agent in Gram stains or cultures of sputum (10).

The author conducted a survey to determine contemporary practice in the examination of lower respiratory tract secretions in 27 leading microbiology laboratories (Figure 2-2). Half provided routine 24 hour service for Gram stains and cultures. The remainder performed these procedures only after approval had been sought. In many laboratories physicians were permitted to perform Gram stains and plant cultures themselves. Although one laboratory performed routine anaerobic as well as aerobic cultures on sputums, half of the respondents indicated that this procedure would not be performed on this type of specimen. The majority of the bacterial flora of the oropharynx consists of anaerobes. Their mixture with indigenous or colonizing facultatively aerobic bacteria yields massively mixed cultures that are nearly impossible to interpret when incubated anaerobically and yield no useful clinical information.

Most microbiologists and laboratory technicians complain that poor quality occurs more commonly among sputums than with any other type of specimen. Most of the respondents in the survey indicated that such specimens were refused and new cultures requested. It was interesting to observe that three laboratories reported refusing over 500 specimens of this type per year and that the overall rate of rejection represented between 2 and 8% of all lower respiratory tract specimens received.

The survey revealed that about 5% of all respiratory tract specimens represented duplicates, that is, more than one specimen received from the same site on the same patient on the same day. Many respondents indicated that they would call the physician or nurse to determine which specimen should be handled; others indicated that only one would be processed and the other would be reported in a manner similiar to a report used in our laboratory stating "See results of duplicate specimen received." Six of the respondents indicated that they would not consider such a report. Three were of the opinion that duplicate specimens *should* be cultured. In the author's laboratory the cumulative report card (see Chapter 4, p. 93) that

Hartford Hospital	Henry Ford Hospital
University California Medical Center	Thomas Jefferson University Hospital
Temple University-Health Science Center	St. Joseph's Hospital
Berkshire Medical Center	University Hospital, University of Washington
Rhode Island Hospital	Wilmington Medical Center
Cleveland Clinic Foundation	Indiana University Medical Center
Hospital for Joint Diseases	Passavant Memorial Hospital
M. D. Anderson Hospital	Jewish Hospital of Saint Louis
Long Island Jewish-Hillside Medical Center	University-McCook Hospital, University of Connecticut
Bronx Lebanon Hospital Center	Yale-New Haven Hospital
Clinical Center National Institutes of Health	Mayo Clinic
Wesley Medical Center	Wadsworth Hospital Center
University of Minnesota Hospitals	Mount Sinai Medical Center
Hospital of the University of Pennsylvania	

Figure 2-2 Laboratories surveyed by the author in a study of procedures for culture of lower respiratory secretions.

is kept on the bench helps to control this problem. This indicates the number of specimens received on a day to day basis. Duplicate specimens are stamped "See results of duplicate specimen received." This reporting system also allows correlation with the previous day's results if daily cultures of lower respiratory tract specimens are being submitted. Eighteen of the 27 laboratories participating in the author's survey indicated that such a correlation with previous work was conducted. It was not clear whether this eliminated unnecessary work. It is certain that this correlation provides guidance to the technologist and minimizes effort for speciation when the same species appear in day to day specimens. This approach might lead to bias and result in misidentification when similar species are confused.

In our laboratory, cultures demonstrating the same gross colonial appearance to that seen on the preceding day are reported "No significant change from previous specimen." This includes spot bile solubility testing of possible colonies of *Streptococcus pneumoniae* and coagulase testing of staphylococcus colonies. There was a difference of opinion among the respondents in the survey regarding this policy. Some thought it risky but desirable; others were against it. Three were issuing such reports. When the same species is isolated from daily sequentially submitted specimens, susceptibility testing is performed in our laboratory only after a 4 day interval. The majority of the respondents subscribed to this approach and repeated susceptibility testing only after a 3–4 day interval. Five did not repeat this test until a 7 day interval had elapsed.

As with all cultures a preliminary report rendered within 18–24 hours is of great value. This makes extra demands on the laboratory clerical force and increases the number of reports processed by nursing stations and entered in the patient's chart. Nevertheless, the isolation of Gram negative rods may have an immediate bearing on treatment and should be reported whenever possible prior to complete speciation and susceptibility testing. Seventeen of the responding laboratories indicated that this was their practice.

Whether the commonly isolated species of *Neisseria, Corynebacteria, Streptococcus viridans*, and *Staphylococcus epidermidis* are reported as such or as "mixed flora" is of little consequence. The majority of the respondents believed that the relative amount of growth on plates was significant enough to report. It is surprising that few laboratories experience requests for Gram stains on more than 10 or 15% of specimens. This may reflect the increasing recognition of the limited diagnostic usefulness of Gram stains. On the other hand, the majority of the respondents believed that Gram stains *were* useful for evaluating infection with *Staphylococcus aureus, Streptococcus pneumoniae*, Gram negative rods, anaerobes, and *Candida sp.* They also agreed that Gram stains are useful for evaluating the quality of the specimen. Although some laboratories placed no limit on the number of potential pathogens that would be "worked up" per culture, it was apparent that most had attempted to place some restrictions on this. In some instances small numbers of colonies would not lead to identification and reporting. Others limited the number of potential pathogens that would be identified to two or three.

Washing or homogenization of lower respiratory tract secretions was not conducted in a majority of the laboratories surveyed. Many proponents of such techniques presented convincing support for these procedures (11). However, the practice of these methods is limited by economics and aesthetics. We believe that the solution to processing specimens contaminated with oropharyngeal material will be found in improved methods of collection.

An objective system for evaluating the quality of lower respiratory tract secretions was established in the author's laboratory. Gram stains are examined under 10X magnification after oil is placed on the slide to improve clarity. The slide is examined for the presence of neutrophils, mucous, and squamous epithelial cells. A rough quantitative estimate is made by applying the scoring system illustrated in Figure 2-3. If the total score is zero or less a report of "oropharyngeal contamination, please repeat" is rendered. Specimens are refrigerated for 72 hours pending any special request for processing.

Specimens with scores of 1–3 are cultured. Complete speciation and susceptibility testing is performed only if the number of potential pathogens isolated does not exceed the score. This arbitrary criterion is based on some very empirical assumptions. Specimens with low scores demonstrate evidence of oropharyngeal contamination and little or no evidence of pyogenic reaction. The probability that potential pathogens, which are isolated, are associated with lower respiratory infection seems remote. Conversely the probability is high that these represent oropharyngeal colonization. These probabilities are reversed when a score of 3 is obtained, signifying the absence of oropharyngeal material and the presence of abundant neutrophils. For over a year in our laboratory specimens yielding numbers of potential pathogens that exceeded the score were reported "potential pathogens isolated—please repeat avoiding oropharyngeal contamination." We now report limited information based on gross colonial morphology of Gram negative rods and spot bile solubility or omniserum testing of alpha hemolytic colonies. This is being done because we had the information and

10–25 neutrophils/10X field	+1
>25 neutrophils/10X field	+2
Mucous	+1
10–25 Squamous cells/10X field	−1
>25 Squamous cells/10X field	−2

Figure 2-3 Criteria for scoring the quality of specimens of lower respiratory secretions.

	Score				
	0	1	2	3	Total
Expectorated	18 (17%)	27 (25%)	34 (31%)	28 (26%)	109
Nasotracheal aspiration	3 (4%)	6 (8%)	15 (20%)	53 (70%)	76
Total	21 (11%)	33 (18%)	49 (27%)	81 (44%)	184

Figure 2–4 Quality distribution of specimens of lower respiratory secretions collected by routine expectoration and nasotracheal aspiration. Quality score is based on Gram stain examination. Note the higher quality of the nasotracheal specimens.

were recording it on the laboratory file slip to correlate with subsequent specimens that might be submitted. We continue to attach a statement indicating oropharyngeal contamination and request a repeat specimen (see Figure 4-2). Clinicians prefer this crude type of bacterial identification to the previous report indicating only that potential pathogens had been isolated. This information could lead to unnecessary or misdirected antimicrobial therapy. Since the previous system gave no clue to the species present in poor specimens, this did not represent a problem.

Specimens from tracheostomy stomata are handled in a similar manner. Secretions taken from the immediate area of the stoma usually show squamous cells from reactive metaplasia localized to the immediate stomal area. Often no leukocytes are present. Potential pathogens isolated from such specimens represent stomal area colonization. Repeats are suggested. Personnel are instructed to obtain secretions from deeper in the tracheobronchial tree. Isolation of potential pathogens from this area correlates more closely with infection. If repeat specimens are received and demonstrate the same multiple pathogens, these are "worked up" and reported. Rarely, more than three potential pathogens are isolated on a specimen that receives a score of 3. In such instances the physician is contacted for a complete discussion of the problem.

Figure 2-4 demonstrates the higher frequency of good quality specimens obtained by tracheobronchial aspiration in contrast to random sputum specimens. A total of 90% of the tracheobronchial aspirates demonstrated scores of 2 or 3 but only 57% of the sputum specimens were of such high quality. It is possible that the tracheobronchial aspirates were better because they were collected from patients with a higher incidence of acute respiratory tract infection than those from whom expectorated specimens were collected. We have observed innumerable instances, however, in which tracheobronchial aspirates of excellent quality followed the collection of poor quality expectorated specimens.

During a random 1 month period 39 of 184 specimens that contained potential pathogens were rejected by this system (Figure 2-5). Sixty-seven of the 268 potential pathogens isolated from these specimens were in the re-

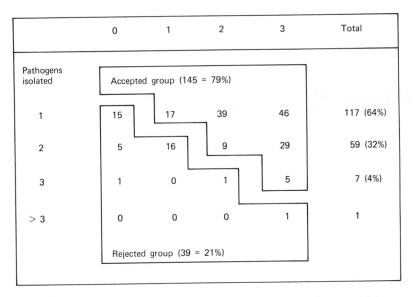

"Q Score"

	0	1	2	3	Total
Pathogens isolated	Accepted group (145 = 79%)				
1	15	17	39	46	117 (64%)
2	5	16	9	29	59 (32%)
3	1	0	1	5	7 (4%)
> 3	0	0	0	1	1
	Rejected group (39 = 21%)				

Figure 2-5 Separation of 184 specimens of lower respiratory secretions containing potential pathogens into accepted and rejected groups based on the score obtained by an examination of the Gram stain. The rejected group contained 67 (25%) of 268 potential pathogens isolated from all specimens. This system eliminates unnecessary laboratory effort and the clinical irrelevance of speciation and susceptibility testing of these isolates from poor quality specimens.

The high quality Q-3 specimen, from which more than three potential pathogens were isolated, was discussed with clinician. He agreed that repeat collection by tracheobronchial aspiration or bronchscopy would be necessary to obtain clinically useful information.

1. Specimens containing potential pathogens
   A. Speciation and susceptibility testing of each potential pathogen   145 ⎱ 184
   B. Rejected with request for repeat because of poor quality   39 ⎰
2. Reported "no significant change from previous specimen" (limited speciation, no susceptibility test performed)   11 ⎱ 55
3. Duplicate specimens (reported as such, not processed)   5 ⎰
4. Mixed flora only (no potential pathogens)   136
5. Sterile   4

Figure 2-6 Disposition of 320 specimens of lower respiratory secretions submitted for culture; 184 (58%) contained potential pathogens. Unnecessary bacteriology was avoided in 55 (28%) because of poor quality, duplication, or evidence of no significant change from a previous specimen submitted within 24 hours.

HARTFORD HOSPITAL

HARTFORD, CONNECTICUT 06115

December 7, 1971

Dear Doctor:

The high incidence of colonization of the upper respiratory tract of hospitalized patients with Staphylococci and various gram negative rods makes it difficult to evaluate the clinical significance of reports of culture of sputum specimens. Lower respiratory secretions should contain a minimum amount of upper respiratory and pharyngeal contamination when submitted for culture. Bronchoscopy produces the best specimens but this is an impractical general solution. Tracheal puncture is being performed more frequently and produces specimens of excellent quality which should be transmitted to the laboratory in the small sterile glass bottles which are used for urine culture.

Tracheal aspiration by Leuken's tube yields specimens of somewhat better quality than the conventional sputum specimen. For some time, we have requested repeat collection by this technique when the Gram stains have suggested poor quality and multiple potential pathogens (excluding D. pneumoniae) have been isolated.

Shortly in the Gram stain sector of the report slip, the letter "Q" will appear followed by a number. 0 to 1 represents very poor quality; repeat specimens will be requested if more than one potential pathogen is isolated. Scores of 2 and 3 represent "fair" to "good" quality. Repeats will be requested on "good" quality specimens only if more than three potential pathogens are isolated. If repeat cultures are of "good" quality and continue to show multiple potential pathogens, those common to both specimens will be reported.

Bacteria and cells observed in Gram stains will be reported on the day received if requested. We believe this is helpful in guiding diagnosis and treatment.

Please consult with us when unusual problems are encountered. This will prevent needless delay which may result when consultations are requested by Dr. Bartlett for specimens associated with unusual or difficult requests. Specimens will be held in the laboratory for 48 hours when consultations or repeat collection is requested.

Sincerely yours,

Raymond C. Bartlett, M.D.
Director
Division of Microbiology

Richard Quintiliani, M.D.
Chief, Infectious Disease
Department of Medicine

RCB:jg

Figure 2-7 Letter sent to the medical staff as part of an educational program to support laboratory efforts to coordinate the quality of specimens of lower respiratory secretions with the extent of bacteriologic evaluation. D. pneumoniae (*S. pneumoniae*) is no longer excluded. Specimens now are stored for 72 hours.

jected group of specimens (Figure 2-6). This represents 25% of the total number of potential pathogens isolated and constitutes a considerable saving of time and expense. It also eliminates the reporting of potentially clinically misleading information.

We have found that personnel, including students, are easily taught to use the scoring system. Random daily checks have demonstrated that scores rarely differ from those obtained by the author or other experienced workers.

Introducing such a program in a community hospital obviously requires the support and cooperation of the medical staff. Educational conferences involving the participation of physicians who are knowledgeable in infectious disease are also essential. Figure 2-7 represents a letter that was distributed to the Hartford Hospital medical staff as part of such an educational program. This program was rapidly accepted by our staff. After 2 years they still support this effort to reduce the confusion that results from reporting multiple potential pathogens and antimicrobial susceptibility data from specimens heavily contaminated with oropharyngeal flora.

MOUTH

Material submitted from different parts of the intestinal tract present unique problems. There is very little that can be done with most specimens that are submitted from the mouth. Cultures of periodontal lesions or saliva usually yield a massively mixed flora of aerobic and anaerobic bacteria. The surgical and antimicrobial approach to therapy in this area presupposes a moderate risk of infection from streptococci and staphylococci. It should not depend on the results of culture from these sites except in unusual situations where collection must be carefully conducted to avoid contamination with indigenous flora. This includes abscesses deep in bone and soft tissues of the maxilla, mandible, face, and neck. Even these will often produce mixed cultures because they derive from sinus tracts or routes of lymphatic transmission of indigenous flora from the oropharynx. A search for *Actinomyces israeili* should always be based on a thorough discussion of the problem between the physician and the microbiologist prior to the collection of material. If this does not occur and isolation of this agent is requested, the microbiologist should hold the specimen and ask for a consultation. Since this organism is indigenous to the mouth, its isolation from material contaminated with oropharyngeal flora is predictable and constitutes a significant waste of laboratory effort.

Physicians should indicate when *Candida* or Vincent's infection is suspected because these are easily recognizable in smears prepared from oropharyngeal material. On the other hand, these agents should not be sought routinely in every specimen submitted from the mouth if this is not specified by the physician. If *Candida* is suspected swab specimens should not be accepted. Instead the physician should be asked to provide curettings which may easily be obtained with a split tongue blade. In oral thrush direct smears demonstrate massive numbers of budding yeasts and pseudohyphae. A culture of *Candida sp.* from the mouth may only indicate colonization and does not establish whether an infection is present.

THROAT AND UPPER RESPIRATORY TRACT

Throat cultures should be incubated anaerobically or in a candle jar to enhance the hemolysis of beta hemolytic streptococci. Reports should only state whether or not Group A streptococcus is isolated. There is some evidence that observation of the relative proportion of streptococcus colonies to normal flora is useful. When beta hemolytic streptococcus colonies represent 10% or less of the total flora the probability of isolating Group A strep is less than 25%. When the majority of colonies represent beta hemolytic streptococci the probability of Group A strep is increased to more than 75%. This finding may be useful for guiding therapy prior to grouping. It is not known whether the proportion of Group A streptococci to normal flora is helpful for separating carriers from infected patients. In areas that are not endemic for diphtheria only health department laboratories should conduct a routine search for these organisms. Similarly, the carriage of *Neisseria meningitidis* cannnot be routinely sought in throat specimens. *Staphylococcus aureus* frequently is isolated from the throats of patients with severe tonsillitis and both viral and streptococcal pharyngitis. Although this organism may cause peritonsillar abscess, its isolation from the throat does not establish a diagnosis of infection.

Extensive bacteriology performed on throat cultures constitutes a significant waste of effort in many of the nation's microbiology laboratories. Many physicians expect isolation of Gram negative rods including *Hemophilus sp.* and *Staphylococcus aureus* to be reported from such specimens. It is widely acknowledged that colonization of the throat with *Staphylococcus aureus* increases in frequency when viral pharyngitis is present. Colonization with this organism and various Gram negative rods increases with the extent of debilitation and the duration of hospitalization. Although aspiration of these bacteria contributes to the development of pneumonia, primary infection of the throat caused by these bacteria is not recognized. (This does not include the specific entity of acute epiglottis caused by *Hemophilus influenzae*. Strictly speaking, this is not a throat infection and when suspected it should be clearly specified on the request slip).

Many pediatricians culture the nose and throat of children to obtain an indirect impression of possible etiologic agents for pneumonia and otitis media because it is difficult to culture the primary site. Both of these infections are acquired from bacterial flora that colonize the nose and throat.

Therefore, it is increasingly doubtful whether a nose or throat culture contributes to the diagnosis and treatment of these infections (12). Predominance of *Streptococcus pneumoniae, Hemophilus influenzae* type B, *Staphylococcus aureus,* or various Gram negative rods in *nose* cultures may be reported because they have some correlation with sinus infection. Patients with chronic allergic rhinitis may demonstrate *Klebsiella ozaenae* which should be reported if it is isolated.

EAR

Specimens submitted for culture from the ear usually represent material draining through a perforated ear drum associated with an acute or chronic infection. In either case direct examination of Gram stains is extremely helpful for establishing whether the material consists of purulent exudate or desquamated material from the external auditory canal. In the latter case mixed flora of cutaneous, upper respiratory, and intestinal types may be isolated and should be reported as such without species identification. An exception is *Pseudomonas aeruginosa* which produces a chronic otitis externa. Masses of hyphae may be observed suggesting *Aspergillus*; this is easily confirmed by a culture. Associated bacteria need not be individually speciated.

Acute pyogenic exudates usually demonstrate a single or clearly predominating organism which should be identified and reported. With increasing chronicity the appearance of Gram negative rods occurs, often in mixed culture. When more than three potential pathogens are isolated from such specimens, it is more helpful to the physician to indicate that a mixed culture has occurred and to request the careful collection of another specimen, preceded by cleansing of the auditory canal to reduce contamination with colonizing bacteria.

Swab cultures of the external canal of newborns may demonstrate neutrophils and bacteria associated with antenatal infection. A Gram stain of this material is useful for the emergency evaluation of sepsis in newborn infants (13).

EYE

Specimens from the eye often reveal one or two potential pathogens which may be isolated and reported. *Neisseria gonorrhoeae* and *Neisseria meningitidis* should be sought in all specimens since they may cause infections at this site in patients of all ages. *Hemophilus sp.* demonstrating X and V dependency but not agglutinating or demonstrating quellung with type B antiserum may represent *Hemophilus aegyptius*. These should be reported only as

Hemophilus sp. because they may represent colonization with other species of *Hemophilus* that are unassociated with conjunctivitis. If *Corynebacterium sp.* are isolated, tests for identification of *Corynebacterium xerosis* should be conducted. Single Gram negative rod species of the enteric type may be reported but multiple isolates of this type usually represent contamination or colonization associated with facial trauma, surgery, or debilitating conditions. Here, identification and sensitivity testing of more than one species should not be performed. *Pseudomonas aeruginosa* may produce an acute conjunctivitis with corneal ulceration and should be reported promptly if observed. *Bacillus sp.* usually represent contamination when isolated from wound cultures. The eye may become infected with this organism, especially when it is introduced through trauma or intraocular surgery. Isolation of *Bacillus sp.* from the eye should not be construed as evidence of contamination and should be promptly reported. Innumerable fungi of marginal human pathogenicity have been associated with infections of the globe. If these are isolated from two or more consecutive specimens the matter should be discussed with the physician.

INTESTINAL TRACT

Specimens of gastric material are sometimes submitted for culture. If the age of the patient is not given, a consultation should be requested. In newborns the presence of neutrophils and bacteria in gastric fluid has been associated with antenatal infection which may have led to pneumonia and generalized sepsis (14). Examining the Gram stain and culture may reveal the etiologic agent. Although patients may swallow mucous that contains the etiologic agents of pulmonary infection, examining gastric contents for material other than fungi and mycobacteria has not been established as a useful procedure. Quantitative studies of the bacterial flora of the stomach or of blind duodenal loops may be significant in patients who have pyloric obstruction or who have undergone gastrojejunostomy (15). This should not be conducted unless techniques are well standardized, clincans are entirely familiar with the interpretation of results, and frequent examinations of this type are to be conducted.

Surgeons frequently submit swab cultures of the stomach and other portions of the intestinal tract at the time of surgery. This is based on a common assumption that postoperative infection is most likely to result from bacteria that predominate in cultures taken at the time of surgery. We perform direct aerobic and anaerobic cultures on such specimens and report a single predominating species. If the culture is mixed, without predominating species, it is reported "mixed intestinal flora." Cultures taken of bowel were correlated with cultures of wound infections taken subsequently from 27 patients at Hartford Hospital. There was agreement in 17 instances. In nine of these a single species was isolated from the wound; in eight cases more than one species was isolated from the wound but one of these was the same as had been isolated from bowel. In six cases sterile bowel cultures were followed by wound infection. In five there was disagreement between isolates from bowel and wound infections. *Escherichia coli, Streptococcus fecalis,* and *Bacteroides sp.* constituted 15 of the 23 species isolated from the 27 patients. Many authorities believe that infection with these species could be predicted allowing accurate direction of antimicrobial therapy without such cultures. It is not practical or clinically useful to report all of the species that can often be isolated from such specimens. If cultures are mixed, with or without a predominating isolate, this should be reported. Following intestinal antibiotic bowel preparation numerous species may still be found in reduced numbers. To provide any idea of predominating species both aerobic and anaerobic cultures must be conducted. Anaerobes predominate at least 50% of the time and often increase relative to aerobes after preparation of the bowel with nonabsorbable aminoglycoside antibiotics which are ineffective against anaerobes.

Cultures of ileostomy or colostomy stomata are sometimes collected when improper healing is observed by physicians. Other than a search for the usual intestinal pathogens the speciation and reporting of various intestinal flora is of no clinical value. Cultures are often submitted from poorly healing wounds surrounding such stomata and are almost always contaminated or infected with aerobic and anaerobic intestinal flora. Unless one or two predominating species are apparent these should be reported as mixed. Examining the Gram stain usually demonstrates whether one is dealing with a purulent exudate from an infected wound or gross intestinal contamination. A similar problem is encountered with material submitted from sinuses or surgical drains. If Gram stains demonstrate massive mixtures of intestinal organisms and cultures grow mixed aerobic and anaerobic flora, they should be reported as such without speciation.

Frequently cultures are submitted from perirectal abscesses. These are almost always mixed and should be reported as such unless one or two predominating species are apparent. A routine search for *Neisseria gonorrhoeae* in all rectal cultures is unnecessary. Clinicians are reminded that suspicion of this organism from this site should be noted on the request slip. On the other hand, when rectal cultures are received with cultures of urethra, vagina, or cervix, laboratory personnel should be instructed to assume that *Neisseria gonorrhoeae* is being sought and inoculate Martin-Lester or Thayer-Martin plates.

When intestinal pathogens such as staphylococci, enteropathogenic *Escherichia coli, Salmonella,* and *Shigella* are suspected, it is useful to indicate that after three specimens are received a consultation is required before additional numbers can be processed. Otherwise there is some risk that innumerable specimens will be received. Reported data indicates that a maximum number of carriers is detected by culture of three consecutive specimens (16). It is doubtful that collecting more than this number will increase the detection of acute infections due to these agents. Examining rectal swabs for intestinal pathogens is a useful and often neglected procedure. Selection of mucopurulent material is important for optimal sensitivity in preparing Gram stains and cultures. Gram stained or Wright stained smears are useful for evaluating the presence of neutrophils which, if increased, may signify any of the bacterial types of enteritis. The presence of mononuculear cells may suggest amoebic infection or viral enteritis. Marked depression of bacterial flora should be reported if observed. This alerts the clinician to the increasing risk of superinfection with *Staphylococcus aureus* or *Candida*. It may also explain the presence of diarrhea in the absence of a specific pathogen. Obvious clumps of Gram positive cocci suggesting staphylococcal enteritis should be promptly reported by telephone. Some Gram positive cocci are seen in most stool specimens and inexperienced technologists often have difficulty determining what is a reportable number.

Technologists and microbiologists sometimes question whether species isolated in pure culture or predominant among normal intestinal flora should be reported when they do not represent established intestinal pathogens. There is some evidence that *Proteus vulgaris* can produce enteritis (17). *Pseudomonas aeruginosa* has produced fatal outbreaks of gastroenteritis in newborns and often colonizes the intestinal tract of patients receiving prolonged courses of antibiotic therapy. Many patients with suppressed normal flora have diarrhea and isolation of predominating species is only coincidental. We report species that predominate over the usual coliforms with the relative amount of coliform flora isolated. There is no longer any justification for assuming that late lactose fermenting variants of various *Enterobacteriaceae*, formally designated "Paracolon species," should be routinely sought in patients with enteritis. A search for an unusual bacterial etiology for unexplained diarrhea should be conducted only after a consultation with the patient's physician. Special techniques may be used for isolating and identifying agents such as *Yersinia enterocolitica, Vibrio parahemolyticus*, and strains of normal intestinal flora that have been implicated in enteritis (17).

URINARY TRACT

No attempt will be made to review the fundamental clinical-microbiologic correlations that have been established for the evaluation of bacteriuria (18). However, many misconceptions of these correlations have developed and these deserve some discussion. The most common error is the assumption that colony counts of less then 100,000 bacteria per milliliter exclude infection and are "not significant." During therapy it is common for bacterial counts to fall into the range between 10,000 and 100,000. For this reason sensitivity testing should always be performed on isolates obtained in this range. Stamey found that one third of urinary tract infections were associated with counts below 100,000 bacteria per milliliter (15). In males a small number of specimens (3%) have been shown to contain more than 10^5 bacteria per milliliter when urine collected suprapubically was sterile. In females a larger percentage (10%) of counts greater than 10^5 per milliliter were associated with sterile suprapubic bladder urine (19). When less than 10,000 bacteria per milliliter are isolated the probability of contamination is significantly large. For this reason incomplete speciation and omission of sensitivity testing is justifiable. If repeated cultures demonstrate the same species in these numbers both the clinician and the microbiologist should recognize the potential clinical significance and agree to complete speciation and antimicrobial susceptibility testing. In many of these instances, patients have long term indwelling catheterization, or neoplasms and fistulas involving the bladder. Treatment of these low grade mixed infections is often futile. If patients develop bacteremia the report may become useful for initiating therapy.

There are many techniques for performing quantitative urine culture. Most of these fail to detect bacteria when less than 1000 per milliliter are present. Several reports have demonstrated that counts below 1000 per milliliter are obtained in a small number of infections. It must be recognized that the current standards for interpreting quantitative urine cultures are based on clean catch urine specimens which are associated with a certain amount of contamination and delay in transmission to the laboratory. It is not appropriate to apply these standards to urine specimens collected by suprapubic puncture or catheterization. Catheterization has been condemned because of the frequency of urinary tract infection that results from this procedure. On the other hand, it does produce specimens in which pure cultures are often found, sometimes with relatively low counts. Therefore, in instances of suspected infection of the urinary tract where cultures fail to produce growth, it may be desirable to inoculate 0.01 ml of urine that has been collected very carefully by catheterization with minimum delay in transmission. It is the practice in our laboratory to speciate and perform susceptibility testing on isolates obtained from these specimens when more than 100 colonies per milliliter are found. When suprapubic puncture specimens are received about 1 ml is placed in thioglycollate broth. If no growth occurs in the quantitative culture containing 0.01 ml, pure cultures obtained from broth are identified and tested for susceptibility. These are reported as 1–100 per milliliter.

Earlier in this chapter the importance of proper collection and transmission of urine specimens was emphasized. If the time of collection is not given, or a delay of more than 1 hour occurs in transmission, we request

Urine specimens not cultured		
Received after delay	20	
Duplicate	1	22
Lab error	1	
Urine specimens cultured		
Sterile		77
Growth		
One isolate	32	
Two isolates	9	45
Three or more isolates	4	
<10,000	7	
10,000–100,000	6	
>100,000	28	
Total specimens received		144

Figure 2-8 Twenty (14%) of 144 urine specimens submitted for culture were reported as "received after prolonged delay." Seventy-seven (63%) of those cultured were sterile. Thirty-two contained only one isolate (71% of 45 cultures showing growth). Four containing three or more isolates were reported as "mixed culture, probable contamination, please repeat."

repeat specimens. In 1 month, during which the nursing service experienced unusual difficulty maintaining these standards, over 200 specimens representing almost 20% of all urine cultures were refused. Recently 97% of the specimens were being received within 2 hours. Some have proposed collecting and transmitting urine specimens for culture by a team specially trained and supervised by the laboratory. Undoubtedly this would add new expense along with scores of other proposals intended to improve patient care. Unless this could improve our current record of 63% sterile specimens and 22% containing only one species, it would not seem justifiable (Figure 2-8). A variety of new techniques employing direct inoculation of the urine at the bedside have been described (21, 22). These utilize slides, patented plastic devices, and pipettes. The cost, correlation with standard methods, and practicality of this approach have been insufficiently studied to indicate that they represent a reliable and economical solution to the problem. An approach utilizing agents that arrest the growth of bacteria during transit has been described but not substantiated by confirmatory reports (23).

The percentage of specimens that are sterile or that contain only one potential pathogen provides a useful index to the care with which specimens are collected and transmitted. The probability exceeds 90% that specimens containing three or more potential pathogens represent contamination. We request repeats on such specimens. These data are summarized in Figure 2-8.

The significance of anaerobic bacteria in the urinary tract is a subject of current controversy. Reports of surveys in which anaerobic culture of urine has been conducted have revealed few, if any, instances of anaerobic infection (24). In one recent report anaerobes were isolated in a small number of patients by suprapubic aspiration (25). A controlled study using collection by suprapubic puncture showed that these agents were absent from the bladder urine prior to catheterization. This suggests that anaerobes are derived from urethral flora and may be introduced into the bladder during catheterization. There seems to be no justification for the routine use of thioglycollate broth, as is the practice in some laboratories. Whether anaerobes or aerobes are isolated this provides no quantification.

GENITAL TRACT

No attempt is made here to review the sensitivity and specificity of various methods for isolation and identification of *Neisseria gonorrhoeae*. It is often difficult to determine from the labeling of a specimen whether a physician is considering gonococcal infection. When rectal cultures are received with urethral exudate a search for *Neisseria gonorrhoeae* is routinely conducted. Specimens of the vagina and cervix from the Emergency Room or outpatient clinics may be from suspected cases of gonorrhea, patients with vaginitis or cervical exudate, which may be associated with endometritis. Selective techniques are again applied for the isolation of *Neisseria gonorrhoeae*.

Practically all specimens of vaginal secretion submitted from in-patients relate to surgical procedures. For this reason we have not routinely sought *Neisseria gonorrhoeae* in such specimens. We have repeatedly advised house staff and attending staff to specify a search for *Neisseria gonorrhoeae* in specimens collected from hospitalized patients in whom infection with this agent is suspected. Increasing interest in the detection of gonorrhea should cause laboratory directors to reevaluate the cost increase that a routine search for *Neisseria gonorrhoeae* in these specimens would incur and relate this to other priorities for the use of laboratory resources. A classic oversight is the physician's failure to request isolation of *Neisseria gonorrhoeae* from specimens submitted from tubal abscesses. These are received so infrequently by the laboratory that technologists cannot be expected to remember that this type of specimen should be cultured for *Neisseria gonorrhoeae*.

Multiple species of bacteria are present in the vagina. These consist largely of intestinal flora with the addition of lactobacilli. When specimens are received from this site, the laboratory worker usually does not know whether the patient has a nonspecific vaginitis or a surgical wound. If vaginitis is stated on the requisition slip the only species that should be sought and reported in mixed culture are group A and B beta hemolytic streptococci, *Corynebacterium vaginale, Candida sp.,* or *Trichomonas.* Others such as *Staphylococcus sp., Corynebacteria* (other than *Corynebacterium vaginale*), nonhemolytic streptococci, lactobacilli, and enterobacteriacaeae should be reported as "mixed vaginal flora" or "mixed intestinal flora."

If it is not stated whether the clinical problem is vaginitis or wound infection we treat the specimen in much the same manner as is described in the section on wounds (p. 16). Lactobacilli, nongroup A, B, or D streptococci, *Corynebacterium* other than *C. vaginale,* and *Staphylococcus epidermidis* are reported collectively as "mixed vaginal flora." When more than two potential pathogens are isolated in addition to the vaginal flora, it is discussed on daily laboratory rounds with the author. Most of them are reported as "mixed vaginal and/or intestinal flora." A trial of evaluation of vaginal specimens by the scoring technique described for wounds (see p. 19) in which Gram stains are examined when the specimen is received has suggested that substantial numbers could be reported as superficial material without evidence of inflammation with request for a repeat collection or consultation regarding planting. When specimens show neutrophils in the Gram stain an effort is made to correlate species suggested by the Gram stain with those that have been isolated to reduce the microbiologic effort and improve the clinical relevance of the report. When this fails to focus attention on one or two isolates, the physician is called for a complete review of the matter. Invariably this results in reporting of the culture as "mixed" with agreement to submit subsequently more carefully collected material.

Cervical specimens from outpatients are cultured for *Neisseria gonorrhoeae.* This is not done on specimens from inpatients in our laboratory for the reasons previously described in the discussion of vaginal specimens. Possible intrauterine infection with a variety of aerobic and anaerobic species is assumed when cervical specimens are submitted. Physicians should request anaerobic cultures if they are not routinely conducted by the laboratory on specimens from this site. Unfortunately secretions from the endocervical canal are frequently contaminated with vaginal flora. We apply the same criteria for evaluation of these specimens as were described above for vaginal wounds and wounds in general.

Evaluating cultures from this area is comparable to examining sputum for etiologic agents of pneumonitis when the specimen has passed through a region in which all of the etiologic agents are either indigenous or frequent colonizers. In the presence of such contamination, reporting one or two predominating species gives no assurance that they represent etiologic agents of intrauterine infection. Techniques for the instrumentation of the endocervical canal have been described (26) but they are inconvenient to use. Physicians also worry about introducing contamination into the endometrial cavity through instrumentation. The need to avoid such confusion is exemplified by the isolation of *Clostridium perfringens* from the cervix. Clinicians recognize the grave prognostic implication of endometritis caused by this organism. On the other hand, the agent is a common component of the vaginal flora and may be easily introduced into specimens collected from the cervical os.

INFECTION CONTROL

Relevance to infection control of cultures collected from the animate or inanimate environment is an important consideration in controlling unnecessary work in some hospitals. We have observed numerous hospitals in which an extensive routine environmental culturing program had been established because of a misconception that this was the most important element of an infection control program, or would at least meet accreditation requirements for such a program. In such cases cultures are often collected by random unstandardized techniques to solve problems that are frequently nonexistant or imagined by those with little experience in the detection and control of hospital infections. When specimens of this type are received by the laboratory they should be brought to the attention of the nurse epidemiologist, or chairman of the infection control committee for an investigation of the source and nature of the circumstances that resulted in the request.

A common pitfall is the infection control committee's decision to collect culture data when specific standards for interpretation of the results have not been established. Even if standard methods are used and methods of interpretation have been reviewed, infection committees often fail to establish whether the information *can be* used productively. We have observed a number of institutions in which a wide range of floor sampling values had been collected over a period of years. Results often indicated undesirably elevated levels of contamination. In some cases no effort had been made to correct the condition and in others these efforts were unsuccessful in bringing about any change in institutional practices. If the infection committee cannot obtain a commitment from the hospital administration to improve maintenance or personnel practices and policies, on the basis of such observations, a culture program represents a waste of time and materials.

The routine culturing of dietary service employees and job applicants for intestinal pathogens is considered useful in many institutions. The frequency of carriers is low enough to permit the assignment of those who are detected to other tasks in the institution where they do not handle food. Some hospitals have established the practice of culturing all prospective nursing employees for *Staphylococcus aureus*. These institutions either refuse employment or treat positive carriers with topical antimicrobials and consider the carrier state irradicated when a reculture is negative. Many of these individuals revert to a positive carrier state. The carrier rate among hospital personnel for this organism is approximately 30% but twice that number may be carriers at one time or another. Intermittant carriers may be missed by a single culture at the time of preemployment physical examination. It is widely acknowledged that no practical means is available to exclude the carriage of *Staphylococcus aureus* by significant numbers of hospital personnel. In the absence of clusters or outbreaks of infection, detection and control measures are not indicated.

If an increase in nosocomial infections suggests a source among personnel, interviews should be conducted to inform workers of the nature of the problem, discuss any recent infections, and collect appropriate cultures. The kinds of cultures collected depends on the type of infection. Staphylococcal carrier states should be sought by culture of the anterior nares. Stools may be collected to detect carriers of intestinal pathogens. Anal and throat carriers of beta hemolytic streptococci have been recognized.

Infection control programs should establish a budget to identify cost for performing cultures or speciation and for typing procedures specifically conducted for surveillance purposes. The laboratory should not be required to subsidize this activity. It will help to draw attention to the cost of extensive surveillance activities. A more complete review of the author's views on the laboratory's role in the surveillance and control of hospital associated infections appears elsewhere (27).

CHAPTER 3

Standardization
of Policies
and Procedures

PROCEDURE MANUALS

Conrad V. Hayes directed the microbiology laboratories at Hartford Hospital for more than 30 years. A self-taught bacteriologist who introduced the author to this clinical science, he enjoyed the extraordinary respect of both clinicians and laboratory workers. He once pronounced that a procedure book could *never* be written about bacteriology. No other activity in the clinical laboratory can compare to the daily bacteriological ritual of deciding how to handle specimens and to interpret results that appear to have no precedent. Someone must always bear the responsibility of running these unique situations through mental permutations, making use of years of experience, and arriving at a decision that could never be anticipated in the preparation of a laboratory manual. Preoccupation with this apparent obstacle causes us to ignore many basic daily decisions that we expect subordinate personnel to make in situations that *can* be anticipated.

Let us establish that procedure books are primarily intended for the inexperienced technician and student (Figure 3-1). A better document would result if we asked these people to list the problems they encounter and make these the substance of a procedure book. Instead the responsibility falls on the supervisor or microbiologist who overlooks these elementary matters and becomes discouraged because he cannot set down in words solutions to all of the various problems brought to his attention.

Procedure book	90%
Updated	45%
Available to personnel	88%
Used by personnel	67%

Figure 3-1   Procedure book status in 100 microbiology laboratories. Although most laboratories had a procedure book in microbiology, most were obsolete and often not used by personnel.

There are many aspects of microbiology laboratory practice that resemble other laboratory areas, such as clinical chemistry, where the preparation of procedure manuals is not so complicated a problem. Reagents, stains, serological, analytical, and staining procedures lend themselves to a simple systematic description. The availability of tests during nights and weekends, proper containers, and methods of planting are the subjects most frequently discussed in bacteriology procedure books.

Experienced workers in small laboratories who perform all the microbiological functions, often with no subordinate personnel, have questioned the need for a procedure book. There is no doubt that procedure books are most valuable in large laboratories where consistent practices must be established among persons of diverse experience and training. The professional who works alone makes many of the same basic everyday laboratory decisions that subordinate workers make in larger laboratories. The process of thinking about each determination during the preparation of a procedure manual would help to provide a uniform approach to many frequently occurring situations. It would also eliminate multiple standards of practice for work performed on specimens from different physicians. Such a handbook would be available to other workers who may be called on to work at night or during periods of sickness and vacation and physicians who may wish to see a statement of policy. Written procedures that contain references to published data supporting a laboratory policy, such as refusal to accept clean catch urine cultures received after a 2–4 hour delay, would be extremely helpful in supporting the position of the microbiologist in a small laboratory where an undocumented policy might be disputed by physicians.

Planting	83%
Collection, transport specimens	62%
Nomenclature	58%
Minimum criteria for identification	57%
Microbiologic precautions	55%
Procedures, materials, quality control criteria	36%
Safety, disinfection, fire	30%
Responsibilities of personnel	28%
Limits on duplicates	26%

Figure 3-2   Procedure book content in 100 microbiology laboratories. Guidelines for planting, collection, and transport have usually been included in microbiology procedure manuals. Quality control, precautions, and safety have been neglected.

Finally, there are third party investigators who require a written document. Most laboratories are under the influence of federal and state regulations which require procedure books. These are mentioned last because they should not be looked upon as the primary reason for developing a procedure book.

The author observed a number of pitfalls while reviewing the use of procedure books in over 100 microbiology laboratories (Figure 3-2). Obsolescence leads to disuse. After the first few times that a worker is told to depart from the written procedure, a progressive disregard for standardization ensues. Gradually the remainder of the book's content fails to reflect actual laboratory practice. Anticipating the amount of effort required for revision is likely to cause further neglect. The first time that a procedure book is written everyone usually "pitches in" with enthusiasm, anxious to see the neatly typed finished product. The revision of an obsolete manual, however, is a rather discouraging chore. This trap can be avoided only by systematically monitoring the manual. This can be incorporated into the routine surveillance of all aspects of the laboratory's operation in a quality control program (see Chapter 6).

Another common pitfall is the publication of criteria for collecting and transmitting specimens in nursing service manuals. A double set of standards is thus developed, creating institutional confusion as the laboratory independently modifies the criteria. Conversely, material contained in some laboratory manuals regarding proper collection, transmission, and availability of tests during nights and on holidays is unavailable and unknown to the medical and nursing staff.

Two other errors have been observed in laboratories where extensive procedure manuals have been written. In the author's laboratory, over a period of 5 years, annual revision eventually led to a massive document containing over 350 pages. Although this contained an abundance of sophisticated criteria for the identification of species of *Aeromonas, Yersinia*, noncholera vibrios, and innumerable nonfermentative Gram negative rods, it did not specify the *minimum* criteria required for identifying *Escherichia coli*, a decision being made between 10 and 15 times per day. This experience led to an entirely fresh approach, which is discussed in the remainder of this chapter. We anticipate that the tendency to include encyclopedic amounts of reference data and to neglect basic everyday laboratory policy will occur in many other laboratories that attempt to develop procedure manuals.

ORGANIZATION OF PROCEDURE MANUALS

Regardless of the size of the laboratory the procedure book should not be looked upon as a single bound document. It will become apparent that organizing the material in subdivided manuals allows convenient distribution of portions relevant to nursing personnel, students, media room personnel, and others. Otherwise one is forced to duplicate certain portions of an intact manual, discard unnecessary sections, or issue entire manuals to those who only require small portions of it. For those who do make use of the entire document, all subdivisions should be bound together. A loose leaf or spiral binding format is preferred, since this allows easy revision and makes books lie flat on the bench when in use. A numbering system should be provided that accommodates the insertion of additional pages or procedures without upsetting an index or table of contents. For example, if the entire document is to consist of six sections, the first might be labeled Pages 1–99, the second, Pages 100–199, and the sixth, Pages 500–599. Furthermore, there should be a gap of several numbers between each procedure or topic to permit the insertion of supplementary pages or of additional topics without being forced to use inconvenient systems, such as, Page 14.1, 14.2, 14A, or 14B. The original document may be typed on pages with copper reinforcements or placed in plastic protectors although the latter produces more bulk. Even in a small laboratory, a clean master copy should be kept in a desk and photostatic copies prepared for laboratory use. Corrections may be entered on the original. This allows additional copies to be made without reproducing pages that are dog-eared, stained, torn, or contain irrelevant handwritten notes.

The preparation of the manual should involve all laboratory personnel. This expedites the work and provides a subtle form of education for everyone. As previously stated, regular surveillance of the manual must be established. This responsibility can be distributed among the original authors. Otherwise obsolescence will soon occur and a major revision is much more difficult than progressively updating the document. It is essential that someone maintain editorial control over the format and organization. Experience has shown that the greatest single problem is to prevent the inclusion of excessive detailed academic material which ignores everyday problems and decisions. In the course of meetings, workshops, and correspondence the author has been requested to provide copies of the Hartford Hospital laboratory procedure book. Although we are glad to provide copies of specific procedures, the cost of reproduction does not permit the distribution of larger portions. Furthermore, the outline provided below should be sufficient to guide laboratory workers in the development of a procedure manual. It is important to review literature and prepare documentation for procedures relevant to each individual institution. Simply copying a procedure from another laboratory excludes the choice of alternatives and may establish inappropriate standards.

It is suggested that the manual be subdivided into the following topics, which are reviewed in the remainder of this chapter.

1. Laboratory administration.
2. Hospital services.
3. Information system.
4. Guide to processing bacteriologic specimens.
5. Minimum criteria for identifying bacteria.
6. Reagents, media, and analytical procedures.
7. Quality control.
8. Reference data.

LABORATORY ADMINISTRATION

Responsibilities of Personnel

Personnel are required to perform procedures and adhere to standards as set forth in the manuals. Supervisors should keep a written record of instances in which personnel have failed to comply with standards—and bring them forth at the time of annual merit appraisal. Temporary modifications must always be approved by supervisors. Those assigned the responsibility of monitoring each section enter on the master copy permanent changes in handwritten form and submit these periodically to be retyped to maintain an updated primary document. Emphasis should be placed on basic responsibilities of subordinate technicians and not on supervisors. This concentrates attention on eyeryday matters and prevents entanglement in complex administrative decisions made by supervisors. This section should include a schedule of working hours and coverage of nights, weekends, and holidays. If the performance of various procedures is divided among the technical staff this should be outlined. In a large laboratory any major division of responsibility among supervisors should be included for the orientation of subordinate personnel.

Responsibility is established here for personnel to conduct quality controls described in procedure descriptions and various surveillance activities outlined in the quality control section. Personnel should be held accountable for informing the supervisor, before reporting results on tests that might be affected, of any quality control observation that exceeds standards set forth in descriptions of individual procedures or in the quality control section.

General Procedures

A general description of the need for proper maintenance of surfaces and equipment should be provided. More detailed schedules for the maintenance and monitoring of equipment should appear in the quality control section.

Personnel should be instructed to wash their hands before eating, smoking, and before and after collecting specimens. Smoking, eating, or drinking at any bench containing viable cultures should be prohibited. Discarding chipped glassware is urged to minimize injuries. Fire safety should include turning off Bunsen burners when not in use and storing flammables in metal cabinets. Procedures for reporting a fire and using fire extinguishers should be described. Rather than attempting a complete description of microbiologic techniques, emphasis should be placed on hazards and certain locally standardized procedures. Mouth pipetting of serum or viable cultures should be prohibited. Pipetting techniques that cause bubbling resulting in aerosols should be prevented. The flaming of pipets, mouths of tubes, and bottles is probably unessential to prevent contamination and may waste more time than it is worth. Centrifuging material containing viable bacteria should be performed only in sealed test tube holders. Potentially infected tissues should only be ground or macerated in a safety cabinet. Materials submitted for isolation of mycobacteria should always be processed in a hood properly ventilated to the outside of the building, preferably through an ultrafilter. Lyophilized cultures must always be handled in a cabinet equipped with ultrafiltration or air incineration unless they can be reconstituted without reopening the vial. A suitable disinfectant is available. This should be poured onto surfaces that become contaminated and cleaned up only after 30 minutes or more for adequate disinfection. Required labeling of tubes and glassware is given.

HOSPITAL SERVICES

This section should indicate which specimens are routinely collected by the laboratory, by physicians, and by other personnel, and procedures that require consultation with the microbiologist prior to collection. It should note the hour that specimens will be received for processing in the laboratory, proper methods of collection and transmission, and, in some cases, normal values. Most hospitals provide this information in the form of tables distributed either directly by the laboratory or through Nursing Service. A 3 × 5 card in a flat or rotary file is sometimes used (Figure 3-3). In either case the format must provide easy reference to questions that arise on nursing units. If a card file is used, that portion relating to microbiology should be incorporated into the microbiology procedure book (Figure 3-4). The Table of Contents and the introductory section of the procedure book should refer to this file so that all personnel know that it is the primary reference for availability of laboratory services. Otherwise there is great risk that the laboratory will change its standards for availability of service without acknowledging and correcting the primary reference file.

Established policies are rarely provided in written form for the many

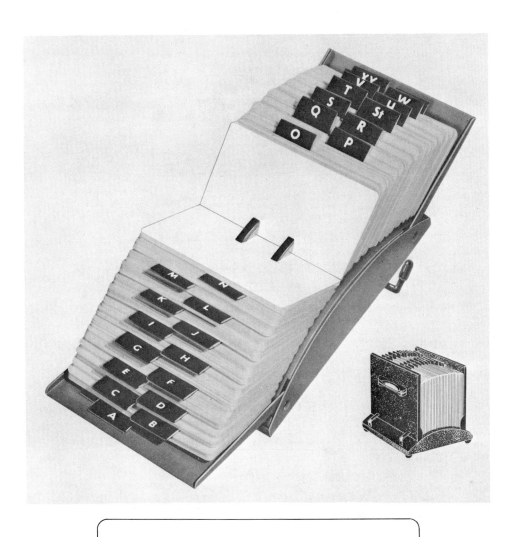

NOSE AND/OR THROAT CULTURE

Requisition Slip: Bacteriology

Container: Swabs placed in tubed Stuart's transport
           media. (Swabs and tubes are available from
           the pharmacy).
Times Available: Cultures are processed from 8 a.m. until
                 10:30 p.m., Monday - Sunday
Time Required for Completion: Cultures are held 24 hours.

Figure 3-3 Rolodex ® file placed on all nursing units for convenient access to information regarding laboratory services (photograph courtesy of Zephyr-American Corp., Long Island City, New York).

```
                                        Card 1
    LABORATORY NIGHT EMERGENCY SERVICE

    Hours:    4 p.m. - 8 a.m., Monday - Friday
              4 p.m. Saturday - 9 a.m. Sunday
              3 p.m. Sunday - 8 a.m. Monday

    Method of Ordering:  The tests listed below will be
    performed by night technicians:  Call the Laboratory,
    ext. 2871 in advance and stamp time on the requisition
    slip upon delivery of the specimen to the Laboratory.
                       SEE NEXT CARD
```

```
                                        Card 2
    LABORATORY NIGHT EMERGENCY SERVICE(Cont. from Card 1)

        The attending physician desiring procedures other
    than those listed below should confer with the attending
    pathologist on call for authorization.
        The names and telephone numbers of the pathologists
    on call are available in the laboratory.
         House physicians desiring procedures other than those
    listed below should direct their request through the
    attending physician on service for discussion with the
    attending pathologist on call.


                    SEE NEXT CARD
```

```
                                        Card 3
    LABORATORY NIGHT EMERGENCY SERVICE(Cont. from Card 2)

    TESTS:  Bacteriology
            All cultures are received and processed until
            10:30 p.m.  After 10:30 p.m., the following
            cultures will be processed only after the techni-
            cian has been called:Blood cultures, spinal fluid
            cultures and Gram stain, operating room cultures,
            cultures from patients admitted to the hospital
            as emergencies since 6 p.m. If, the technician is
            not called specimens found at 7 a.m. collected
            prior to 3 a.m. or with no collection time given
            will be reported"Received after prolonged delay".
```

Figure 3-4   Cards from Rolodex® file used on nursing units. These indicate the availability of night emergency services in the laboratory and in Bacteriology.

problems that result from improper submission of specimens to the laboratory. What is the policy of the laboratory when a urine culture is delivered at midnight, no one is called, and it is found at 8 a.m.? If it has been clearly stated that urine cultures are not planted after midnight unless the technician is called, medical and nursing staff must be forewarned of the consequences of such a situation (Figures 3-5 and 3-6). If the laboratory has established a written policy not to plant urine cultures that are delayed more than 4 hours what action is taken? Is a written report sent indicating that the specimen was not planted because of excessive delay? Does someone call the nursing staff or the physician? Is the specimen discarded or saved so that it can be planted if there is something irretrievable about it? The lack of a published statement of policy on these matters leads to much rancor among physicians, nurses, and laboratory personnel. Anticipation of such conflict frequently causes indecision on the part of laboratory personnel who process poor specimens when new material should be collected.

INFORMATION SYSTEMS

A subsequent chapter deals with the unique information problems that arise in microbiology and the systems that may be applied to control them. Within the administrative section of the procedure book, the responsibilities of personnel in the use of information systems should be described, beginning with criteria for identifying specimens. There must be specific guidelines for handling specimens that are received without proper labeling or identification. Workers should be advised against guessing at the processing of specimens when they do not understand the terminology used to describe the site or type of examination requested. Guidelines for consulting with supervisors and returning such requisitions to their origin for clarification should be provided.

The method of assessioning should be described. This should include identifying who is responsibile for picking up and processing specimens promptly. If time clocks are used to document these steps this fact should be included. Specify the information to be entered in the laboratory log, work card, or other assessioning system. In most cases this includes the patient's name, history number, and location. Additional information, such as the date, time of collection, nature of specimen, and procedure requested, may require transcription as well. Personnel should be warned against abbreviating or omitting portions of the request and instructed to record the type of container received if this has a bearing on the interpretation of the specimen. Improper submission or evidence of contamination should also be documented. This section may also include instructions for preparing additional requisition slips to accommodate multiple analyses on specimens. It is always essential to require initialing during the assessioning procedure to

Note 1

     Bacteriology-Conditions affecting processing:
If specimen is found in the lab at 7 a.m. with
    a)   elapse of more than 6 hrs. since collection
or, b)   required time of collection not given; or if
           elapse of time between collection and receiving
           during day exceeds maximum established for
           specimen,-
Specimen will be refrigerated for 72 hours and report
rendered "received after prolonged delay". Physician
should consult with Dr. Bartlett if a fresh specimen
cannot be submitted in its place.

Note 2

     Bacteriology-Conditions affecting processing:
Additional clinical information is required prior to
processing or collecting certain types of specimens.
Preliminary report requesting consultation with
Dr. Bartlett will be rendered. Specimen will be held
72 hours pending such consultation.

Note 3

     Bacteriology-Conditions affecting processing:
Cultures of wounds, urine, mucous membranes and
respiratory secretions will be limited to one per day.
When labeling indicates duplication one specimen will
be reported "See results of duplicate specimen received".
It will be refrigerated for 72 hours pending any consultation between the physician and Dr. Bartlett to justify
processing.

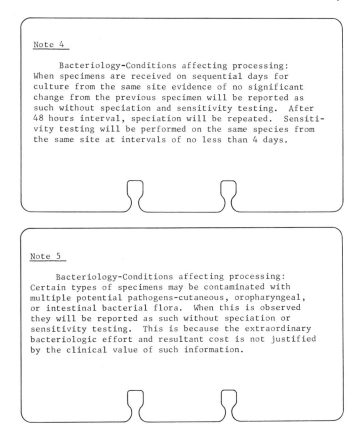

Figure 3-5 Rolodex® cards establishing conditions that affect the processing of bacteriologic specimens. These are on each nursing unit and provide justification for requests for repeat when specimens are improperly submitted.

identify the handler. Instructions should be provided for processing and reporting emergency requests.

Specific criteria for reporting should be established. If preliminary reports are issued, it might be desirable to establish 48 hours as a maximum interval between assessioning and reporting. Reports on direct examinations and other tests performed in Microbiology, such as serologic procedures, must be rendered on the day they are received. All morphologic, biochemical, and serologic observations made during the processing of specimens should be recorded in a systematic and legible fashion. Whatever system is in use, personnel should be provided with specific instructions about the complete and thorough recording of this type of information. The person who has performed these observations should be sure to initial the record.

Use of correct spelling and current nomenclature should be stipulated. Instead of attempting to provide a typed list of all the bacterial species that may be encountered, it should be sufficient to indicate that accepted bac-

SPUTUM AND LOWER RESPIRATORY SECRETIONS FOR CULTURE
                                        Card 1-see Card 2
Requisition slip: Bacteriology #5
Container: Specimens may be collected by the following
means listed in order of increasing probability of provid·
ing good quality material. In all cases irrelevant coloni·
zation should be avoided by rinsing mouth,cleaning trache·
ostomy,stoma,etc. 24 hr. collections or specimens
wrapped in tissues will not be accepted.
     Sputum-paper carton (available from storeroom)
     Tracheal suction-sterile plastic or Leukens tube.
     Bronchial secretions-sterile plastic or Leukens tube.
Amount Needed: 2ml or more
Times available: 8am-10:30pm., Monday-Sunday

SPUTUM AND LOWER RESPIRATORY SECRETIONS FOR CULTURE
                                        Card 2-see Card 3
Time required for completion:
  All sputums are routinely reported after 48 hours.
If "stat" smears are desired, please request them. They
will be reported promptly.

SPUTUM AND LOWER RESPIRATORY SECRETIONS FOR CULTURE
                            Card 3

    Mucous from the lower respiratory tract including
sputum will be examined by Gram stain and classified
from Q-0 to Q-3. Q-0 indicates primarily oropharyngeal
material. Q-3 indicates purulent exudate without oropharyngeal contamination. Limited bacteriology will be
performed on poor specimens and repeats will be requested
if oropharyngeal contamination predominates.

    Lower respiratory secretions for anaerobic cultures
must be collected by bronchial tracheal aspiration free
of pharyngeal contamination.

Figure 3-6 Rolodex® cards provide directions and conditions for proper submission of sputum and lower respiratory secretions for culture.

teriologic nomenclature must be used except where it is otherwise specifically authorized. Thus it is the technician's responsibility to check the proper term or spelling in reference material used in the laboratory. This represents another simple illustration of a factor that can expand and complicate procedure books. There is no need to provide lists of current nomenclature with proper spelling if these are available in textbooks on the laboratory shelf. Consistency in the use of both genus and species names should be established. This also applies to abbreviations of genus and species. If stamps are employed to provide uniformity on this issue, their consistent use must be stipulated.

It would be desirable to provide a section on courtesy in responding to inquiries of persons who enter the laboratory or telephone about specimens and reports. Although it would seem unnecessary, personnel often require guidance in matters of common courtesy. For example, conversation with other workers or processing of specimens should be interrupted. Telephones should not be allowed to ring for extended periods of time and should not be answered with "yes" or "lab" but with some consistent term such as "Microbiology laboratory, may I help you?" Inquirers should not be left waiting for 5 or 10 minutes while information is being sought. Many laboratories have a personnel manual which contains this type of information, as well as acceptable attire, use of radios, and so forth. This approach is preferable to a separate description in procedure books in different divisions of the laboratory, which might result in inconsistent standards.

Recording quality control data is often neglected by technicians. That this is as essential as recording observations on patients' specimens should be emphasized. The same is true of recording work performed on daysheets to provide an accurate accounting of workloads.

Use of Reference Laboratories

Specific instructions should be set forth for submitting specimens to reference laboratories. The proper forms, information to be provided, and maintenance of cultures in a viable state until reports are received should be presented. This also applies to the processing of sera and other materials which may be sent to other laboratories for tests not conducted in some hospitals. If state regulations require the laboratory to report the results of tests that may suggest or establish certain "reportable diseases," instructions for this should be provided.

GUIDE TO PROCESSING BACTERIOLOGIC SPECIMENS

This section provides guidelines for direct examinations, media to be inoculated, conditions of incubation, and inspection and disposition of isolates. Most of this material can be arranged in tabular form. There are sufficient numbers of unique considerations for specimens from various body sites to warrant a narrative of each. These may follow the tables.

The first consideration is whether the specimen has been properly collected and submitted. This was discussed in the previous section (Hospital Services, pp. 50–51). It is best to keep this information separate from tables of instructions for laboratory workers. Otherwise selective transcription for use by nurses and physicians, or providing this portion of the procedure manual to them with irrelevant instructions for laboratory processing of specimens is required. A statement reminding personnel that they are responsible to report to supervisors specimens that are improperly collected and submitted should be sufficient. Any separate reference to these standards here raises the previously mentioned risk (p. 48) of developing double standards.

Tables may be prepared for types of specimens and requests for which consultation between the physician and the microbiologist should be sought prior to processing, direct examinations to be performed, media to be inoculated and conditions of incubation.

Specimens and requests requiring consultation might include the following: (a) requests for nonspecific cultures of the mouth; (b) anaerobic culture of sputum or urine; (c) inanimate environmental; (d) requests for Gram stain on throats or blood; (e) smears for mycobacteria from gastric content or urine; (f) culture of feces or spinal fluid for mycobacteria; (g) processing of more than three specimens for isolation of enteric pathogens or ova and parasites from feces, or isolation of mycobacteria or fungi from any specimen; and (h) culture of fungi from specimens submitted nonspecifically as "fungus culture." Exceptions may be skin and nail scrapings that are examined directly and cultured for *Candida* and dermatophytes, spinal fluid for *Cryptococcus*, blood for yeasts and *Histoplasma*, or vaginal, anal, and oral material for *Candida*. This may be tabulated separately or combined with instructions for direct examinations, culture, and incubation. Elsewhere in the manual detailed instructions are given for handling data, preparing direct examinations, proper use and interpretation of media, methods of microaerophilic, capneic, and anaerobic incubation, and so forth. These need not be expanded upon in this section.

Figure 3-7 illustrates a narrative presentation of information unique to a particular type of specimen. The disposition of isolates from spinal fluid or blood leaves little alternative to speciation and reporting of anything that is isolated. On the other hand, multiple species in disparate proportions are often isolated from lower respiratory secretions and wounds. Some may be considered indigenous normal flora, others are colonizers with pathogenic potential, and yet others may be pathogens. The judicious application of microbiologic effort, in which the resulting cost bears some direct relation to the clinical value of the report, has been thoroughly treated in previous chapters. In the procedure manual the microbiologist must spell out basic instructions which will support such a policy through the actions of inexperienced workers. Will one or both of the terms "mixed flora" or "normal flora" be used? What observations are required of an isolate to assess it as mixed or normal flora? What types of colonies require speciation? If one alpha hemolytic colony is observed in a sputum culture is this worked up to exclude *Streptococcus pneumoniae*? What should be done about one colony of a Gram negative rod? If one colony can be ignored, what about five? If there are five colonies of something that resembles *Klebsiella* and fifty that look like *Escherichia coli,* are both speciated and tested for antimicrobial susceptibility? If a wound contains one Gram negative rod species, this isolate will obviously be speciated and tested for antimicrobial susceptibility. What about two, three, or four species; in equal proportions; in disparate proportions? Every microbiologist knows that his personnel cannot take the time to identify and test the antimicrobial susceptibility of every isolate. It has been repeatedly emphasized that even if sufficient time were available it would be clinically irrelevant or misleading, and unnecessarily expensive. Although every experienced clinical microbiologists knows this, we continue to put inexperienced technologists in the position of determining what to isolate without providing specific criteria to assist them in making these decisions.

MINIMUM CRITERIA FOR IDENTIFYING BACTERIA

Many microbiologists have developed tables and guides to microbial identification for their workers. As previously noted, there has been a tendency in many laboratories to exhaust all available reference material and provide elaborate tables of distinguishing characteristics for the identification of large numbers of species, the majority of which are infrequently isolated (Figure 3-8). At the same time no criteria are given for the minimum number of distinguishing characteristics that must be applied to common isolates, such as *Escherichia coli.* When this organism is submitted as a proficiency testing specimen, agencies receive an exhaustive series of morphologic and biochemical determinations that have absolutely no bearing on the criteria used to identify this organism in daily work. Substantial numbers of highly proficient microbiology laboratories condone the identification of this organism on the basis of gross colonial morphology from selected specimens, such as urine. These limited criteria are supplemented by supportive susceptibility testing results (see p. 99, Chapter 3). However, nowhere in the procedure books of these institutions can this policy be found. The list of species for which minimum identification criteria are established should be limited to isolates that are observed at least once a month (Figure 3-9). Less frequently observed species should be brought to the attention of the microbiologist, who may then draw on reference ma-

RESPIRATORY TRACT SECRETIONS

A.   Laboratory Receiving and Processing

  1.   Conditions affecting processing

      a. Requisitions-requests for pneumocystis will be reported
         "Consultation required for performance of test" and the
         specimen held in the refrigerator for 72 hours.

      b. Quality Requirements-Specimen should consist of mucoid
         material free of salivary secretions. Specimens should
         be stamped out inadequate if the following conditions
         are found: salivary secretions devoid of mucous; less
         than 1 cc of material; improper container; evidence of dry-
         ing.

B.   Planting

  1.   Routine smear and culture

      Note on report card type of specimen: trach, cup sputum,
      leukens, etc. Select mucopurulent portions for processing.
      Prepare Gram stain. Oil slide. Examine under 10X and score
      as below:

$>$10 neutrophils/average field	+1
$>$25 neutrophils/average field	+2
$>$10 squamous cells	-1
$>$25 squamous cells	-2
mucous	+1

      List score in lower right. Gram stain area as Q-1,Q-2,etc.
      If score is Q-0 or less report as Q-0. Do not plant or re-
      port Gram stain results on specimens yielding Q-0 scores.
      Report "Specimen consists primarily of oropharyngeal material,
      please repeat". Refrigerate 72 hours pending any special
      request for processing.

      If score is Q-1 or greater inoculate plates using swab.
      After planting, streak "x" of Staph aureus on BAP. Place media
      in CO_2 incubator. Examine smear for bacteria and cells, if re-
      quisitioned and record results.

C.   Routine culture

      When routine Gram stains are requested, record and return preliminary
      report same day. If requested "stat" report by telephone within one
      hour of receiving specimen.

D.   Anaerobic culture

      If expectorated sputum is submitted report "Please submit material
      collected directly from trachea or bronchi for anaerobic culture".
      Store 72 hours. If proper material is submitted, select purulent
      appearing portion for inoculation of media. Prepare direct smear.
      Inoculate anaerobically 48 hours. Perform aerobic culture if not
      requested.

58

E. Fungus culture

    If unspecified fungus culture is requested stamp "Consultation
    required for performance of test" and store 72 hours.

F. Culture or smear for acid fast bacilli

    (See Mycobacteria Section)

G. Identification and Reporting

    Examine plates for colonies representing Neisseria, Coryne-
    bacteria and non-hemolytic Streptococci. These may be reported
    as mixed flora on colonial morphology; Gram stain if in doubt.

    Isolate, identify and report: when any colonies resembling D.
    pneumoniae, Staph aureus, hemolytic B. streptococci, or H. influenzae
    are observed; when more than five colonies of a Gram negative
    species or micrococcus is observed. Perform coagulase tests on
    colonies resembling Staph aureus or micrococcus colonies: report
    Staph aureus if positive; include with mixed flora if negative.
    Perform spot bile solubility test on colonies suspect of S. viridans
    or D. pneumoniae; report D. pneumoniae if positive; include with
    normal flora if negative; if yeast are isolated in pure culture
    refer to Mycology for speciation; if in mixed culture report yeast.
    If satelitic Hemophilus colonies are observed test with Type A and
    B antisera. If positive report Hemophilus influenzae Type B; if
    negative report Hemophilus species.

    If number of potential pathogens isolated exceeds score, report
    isolates generically without speciation or susceptibility testing,
    suggest repeat avoiding oropharyngeal contamination and hold. If
    repeat specimen is processed and shows same potential pathogens
    but score is exceeded consult supervisor before reporting.

H. Anaerobic cultures

    After two (2) days incubation refer to supervisor for evaluation.
    Have Gram stain available for examination.

RCB 11/72

Figure 3-7 Procedure for processing lower respiratory secretions submitted for culture.
Specific planting instructions are condensed elsewhere in the procedure book. Similarly
minimum criteria for identification of common isolates follows in another section of the
procedure book.

This description contains directions that are unique for lower respiratory secretions. Note
the emphasis on interpreting Gram stain and criteria for reporting colonies of potential
pathogens.

IDENTIFICATION OF KLEBSIELLA-TRIBE KLEBSIELLEAE

The tribe KLEBSIELLEAE is composed of non-motile bacteria conforming to the definitions of the family ENTEROBACTERIACEAE. All genera of the tribe generally have the following key characteristics in common, although rare exceptions do occur with regard to INDOL, MR-VP.

INDOL -	Simmons Citrate +	KCN +
MR -	H_2S (TSI) -	PAD -
VP +	Urease	

Citrate +
Urease (+)d
Arabinose +
Sorbitol +
Malonate +
VP 37° +
VP 22° +
Lysine decarb. +
Ornithine decarb. -
Gelatin (22°) -
Motility -
ONPG +
TSI A/AG

The genus Klebsiella is composed of non-motile bacteria. A summary of key descriptive reactions is shown in the capsule table to the left. The most common specie is K. pneumoniae found in a wide variety of clinical specimens from the respiratory tract to the urinary and intestinal tracts; however, from a historical viewpoint, the organism was originally associated with pneumonia and was commonly referred to as "Friedlanders Bacillus" (after its discoverer). Frequently K. pneumoniae is encapsulated and using specific capsular antiserum isolates may be assigned to designated types based on Quellung reactions. As of 1965 Kaufmann (1966) lists 72 different species of Klebsiella. On TSI Klebsiella pneumoniae is usually indistinguishable from Enterobacter cloacea or E. aerogenes since they all show typical acid slant and acid and gas butts without demonstrable H_2S production. A small % (6%) of K. pneumoniae was found by Edward and Fife (1955) to be Indol positive +, 3.3% liquified gelatin. These variants are sometimes referred to as K. pneumoniae biotype "Oxytoca". Klebsiella rhinoscleromatis and K. ozaenae are rarely encountered clinically; however, they can pose as diagnostic problems by being MR+, VP- and lysine decarboxylase negative. It is conceivable that an isolate from the nose or throat that presents an Alk/A TSI showing small amounts of gas and no H_2S that is citrate negative and ONPG positive will be classified as an E. coli. A negative ornithine and a positive ADONITOL test, plus negative motility would place such an isolate in the Klebsiella group.

Differentiation of species within the genus Klebsiella
(Commonly used biochemical tests)

Test or substrate	K. pneumoniae [1]		K. ozaenae [1]		K. rhinoschleromatis [1]	
	Index	%+ (%+) [2]	Index	%+ (%+) [2]	Index	%+ (%+)
Hydrogen sulfide	-	(4)	-	0	-	0
Urease	+	94.5	d	9.5(10.3)	-	0
Indol	-	94	-	0	-	0
Methyl red 37C	-or+	13.3	+	99.1	+	100
V-P 37C	+	91.1	-	0	-	0
Citrate (Simmons)	+	97.7		31.9(31)		
KCN (growth)	+	97.9	+or-	88	+	100
Motility	-	0	-	0	-	0
Gelatin 22C	-	3.3	-	0	-	0
Lys. decarb.	+	97.2(2.8)	-or+	48	-	0
Arg. dihydro	-	.9	-	6	-	0
Ornithine decarb.	-	0	-	4	-	0
Phenylal.deam.	-	0	-	0	-	0
Glucose:						
acid	+	100	+	100	+	100
gas	+	96.5	d	64(2)	-	0
Lactose	+	98.2(1.4)	d	24.1(70.7)	(+)or-	(72.8)
Sucrose	+	98.9	d	16.3(17.3)	+or-	68.2(31.8)
Mannitol	+	100	+	100	+	100
Dulcitol	-or+	31.5	-	0	-	0
Salicin	+	99.7(.3)	+	97.4(2.6)	+	100
Adonitol:						
acid	+or-	87.7	+	98.3(1.7)	+	100
gas	d	83.4(.3)	d	60(2)	-	0
Inositol						
acid	+	97.9(.8)	d	58.6(21.6)	+	95.5(4.5)
gas	+	91.9(2)	d	28(8)	-	0
Sorbitol	+	99.4(.3)	d	78(10)	+	100
Arabinose	+	99.9	+	100	+	100
Raffinose	+	99.7	+	90	+or (+)	68.2(31.8)
Rhamnose	+	99.3(.4)	d	60(8)	+	95.5(4.5)

Index:
    +, positive within 1 or 2 days' incubation
   (+), positive reaction after 3 or more days
    -, no reaction
  +or-,majority of strains positive, occasional cultures negative
  -or+,majority of cultures negative, occasional strains positive
 (+)or+,majority of reactions delayed, some occur within 1 or 2 days
    d, different reactions: +, (+), -

Numerals in parentheses indicate percentage of delayed reactions (3 or more days)

(Data from CDC)

Figure 3-8 Example of excessively detailed information provided for identification of bacteria. Note that no reference to minimum criteria is provided. Such information may confuse and mislead inexperienced workers. It should be available in the reference section of the manual for use by experienced personnel.

Figure 3-9 Identification table for Gram negative rods

	Day 1		Day 2 — Rapid Proced.													Day 3						
Gross Appear.	Presum. Ident.		TSI Slant	Butt	Gas	Citrate	Indole	Motility	Ornithine	Report	Urea	PAD	ONPG	Oxidase	Typings	Lysine	MR	VP	DNase	Arabin.	Malon.	Report
Acid 4+	E.coli (1)		A	A	S	0	+	+	V	E. coli												
	Coliforms		A	A	S	+	0	+	V	Citrobacter												
Acid 2+	Kleb-Ent.		K	A	0	+	0	0	0	Klebs.pneu.												
	"		K	A	0	+	0	V	+	Enterobact. sp.												
Acid 0	Proteus sp.								+	Proteus mirab.												
Swarms	"								0	Proteus vulg.												
Green	Pseudom.									Ps. aerug.				+								
	Gram neg. rd.																					
	"		K	A	V	+	+	V	O	P.vulgaris	+	+	0									
	"		K	A	V	O	+	V	+	E.coli	0	0	+									
	"		K	A	+	+	O	+	+	Ent.-Serr.	0	0	+						0	+		Enterobacter
	"		K	A	V	+	+	V	O	Gram neg. rd.	0	+	0						+	0		Serratia
	"		K	A	V	+	+	V	O	"	+	+	0									
	"		K	A	V	O	+	V	+	"	+	+	0									
	"		K	A	V	O	O	+	0*	P. rettgeri	0	0	0		(7)	+	+	0			0	
	"		K	A	S	O	+	V	+	P.morgani	0	0	+		(3)	+	0	+				
	"		K	A	S	O	+	+	0*	S.typhi*	0	0	0		(6)	+	+	0			0	
	"		K	A	O	O	+	+	V	Citrobact.	0	0	0									
	"		K	A	O	O	+	O	V	Salm.ent.*	0	0	0	+	(2)	+	+	0				
	"									E. coli												
	"									Gram neg. rd.												
	"		K	A	O	O	O	O	+*	Shig.sonnei*	0	0	0		(4)	0	+	0				
	"		K	A	O	O	V	O	O*	Shig.group*	0	0	0		(5)	0	+	0				
	"		K	O	O	+	O	O	O	Herellea(8)	0	0	0									

(1) urines only: "SEN" must accept
(2) Shigella typings neg; A-D typings (+)
(3) Salmonella neg. Beth-Bal (+)
(4) Pos Shigella group D
(5) Pos Shigella groups A,B,C
(6) Pos Salmonella
(7) Pos Salmonella group D
(8) OF glucose oxidative; OF xylose acid; nitrate neg

(*) Report to supervisor if these results are obtained

Figure 3-9 Minimum tests required for identification are clearly shown with results necesary for identifying common Gram negative rod isolates. This provides basic guidance for inexperienced personnel and establishes a uniform policy. Unusual isolates or problems that are encountered require consultation with experienced workers who are able to use material in the reference section.

terial at his disposal. The emphasis should be placed on guiding the inexperienced worker in the daily decisions that will be made *without* consultation with senior personnel. This minimizes the effort required to prepare this portion of the procedure manual but forces senior personnel to make some fundamental decisions which they may have been avoiding.

The following example of the urgent need for candor on this issue was observed by the author. A technician in a small hospital laboratory performed substandard work in a proficiency survey. She was tutored by specialists in a performance evaluation program who sent her back to work to conduct 24 biochemical tests on every Gram negative rod that she isolated! We were asked to accept overflow work from this laboratory because the technician could not handle the load!

Several years ago the Council on Microbiology of the Commission on Continuing Education of the American Society of Clinical Pathologists was requested to provide a set of minimum criteria acceptable to performance evaluation groups and applicable to all laboratories. Most doubted that such a document would withstand criticism. It was prepared, proved provocative, and is no longer generally available. This experience provided convincing evidence that it is the professional prerogative of every qualified clinical microbiologist to decide what level of confidence is required for microbial identification in his particular laboratory. Public and private performance evaluation groups would like to see uniform standards established. We do not believe that every laboratory in this country qualified to do bacteriology can be locked into the same economic and academic pattern. We must observe, and be prepared to act on, the policies of performance evaluation programs that have gone beyond scoring on the basis of correct identification alone and have begun awarding the greatest number of points to those who report the most exhaustive list of differential criteria. This would be comparable to lauding the intern who orders the largest number of laboratory tests. From an economic point of view the laboratory that gets the *most* clinically useful answers by applying the *smallest* number of criteria should get the most credit.

The author's laboratory was the only one approved for comprehensive mycology in the State of Connecticut to receive half credit on a proficiency test for reporting a *Candida* as "*Candida species*, not albicans" instead of "*Candida tropicalis*." Although infections with *Candida* species other than albicans are well known, there is insufficient diagnostic or therapeutic significance attached to differentiating these species to warrant establishing the capability to conduct such speciation in multiple laboratories within one state. The grading should have been just the reverse, awarding only half credit to those laboratories that exerted unnecessary effort to produce information of no added clinical value.

Thyroglobulin Antibody Test

Place 0.9 ml of sheep cells in tube. Add 0.1 ml

of serum. Mix and let stand 45 minutes. Centrifuge

5 minutes. Place 0.1 ml sensitized sheep cells in each

well in test plate. Add 0.1 ml of supernatant serum from

tube to first well. Serially dilute. Cover plate with

cellophane and rotate 5 minutes. Read after standing

overnight. Positive is flat mat of cells. Negative is

button.

Figure 3-10 Inadequate description of procedure. Note the omission of basic principle; detailed list of materials required; control materials; temperatures; speed of centrifugation; guidelines for reading results; and basic clinical significance.

REAGENTS, MEDIA, AND ANALYTICAL PROCEDURES

A concise format must be established for descriptions of analytical procedures (Figures 3–10 and 3–11). They should provide adequate documentation but avoid excessive supporting information, which can be referred to in the bibliography. Undesired duplication results if all quality control requirements are repeated with each procedure. The *responsibility* of personnel to conduct quality control measures should be stated in the administrative section of the manual. This should also include the action to be taken when control results are unacceptable. The *frequency* with which control measures are conducted and general standards of acceptability that are not unique to individual procedures should be placed in the quality control section. Only those aspects of quality control that are unique for a specific test should be included in the description of that procedure. This eliminates much repetition.

Biochemical tests, anaerobic technique, antimicrobial susceptibility testing, staining, and serological procedures lend themselves to a similar approach. Each description should begin with a *statement of principal* consisting of two or three sentences briefly incorporating the chemical and biological mechanisms involved, the observed reaction which occurs, and its fundamental microbiologic and clinical significance. This should be followed by a *description of materials* required. When preparing this information, imagine that you are submitting a list of materials to be obtained by someone else for performing this procedure in another institution (Figures 3-12 and 3-13).

Always list the grade and source of chemical reagents because substitution of reagents contaminated with impurities or obtained from a different manufacturer may significantly affect the performance of the test. On the other hand, the use of analytical grade reagents may be unnecessarily expensive where lower grades will suffice. Biological reagents require broader specification. If material from a specific manufacturer is reproducible and specific for a particular procedure, it may serve simply to give reference to this source. Otherwise some statement must be made to indicate the expected performance of the product.

The potency and specificity of antigens and antisera presents a special problem. Many polyvalent antisera contain specificity for several bacterial antigens. In addition there may be some nonspecificity for heterologous antigens. A concise description would include the minimum titer of activity against antigens for which specificity is desired and a maximum titer of activity against nonspecific antigens. The same problem applies to commercial antigens. The CDC has established an extensive program for evaluating and testing biological reagents. Many manufacturers voluntarily submit their products for such evaluation. The results are provided to directors of health department laboratories throughout the 50 states who, in turn, transmit this information to hospital laboratory workers upon request. The CDC and eminent laboratory workers throughout the country have urged microbiologists to specify on purchase orders for biological materials that the product must conform to CDC specifications. This does not bind the manufacturer to submit his product to CDC but will cause him to provide control data conforming to these specifications. It is likely that wider stipulation of this requirement on purchase orders would lead to greater use of the CDC evaluation program by manufacturers.

It would greatly simplify procedure descriptions if performance standards for biologic reagents could be defined as "meeting CDC minimum performance standards." The alternative is to spell out the performance characteristics of the reagent in the procedure description. This assumes that someone in the laboratory that performs the procedure must insure that the reagent conforms to the characteristic stated if there is no evidence from the manufacturer, or other independent evaluation, that the product complies with these criteria. It is quite obvious that individual clinical laboratories are not in a position to carry out such extensive evaluation of biological products. Limited surveillance is desirable to guard against contamination and loss of activity; this is discussed in Chapter 6. The important point of this discussion is to draw recognition to the common practice of performing analytical procedures with biological materials of which the specificity and

THYROGLOBULIN ANTIBODY

PRINCIPLE:

To detect antibody to thyroglobulin by agglutination of thyroglobulin sensitized sheep cells. Non-specific sheep cell agglutinins
that may be present in patients' serum are first absorbed by incuba-
ting test serum with "control sheep cells". Following adsorption,
serum is serially diluted with "thyroglobulin sensitized sheep cells".

EQUIPMENT:

1. Plexiglass diluting tray (Intercontinental Scientific Co.,
New York, New York). This tray measures 23 cm. x 18 cm. x 2 cm. There
are 8 rows of 10 wells. Each well has a volume of 2 cc. The wells
are conical with a pinpoint central depression. They measure 2 cm.
across with a central depth of 1.5 cm. The size and shape of the well
are critical; rounded bottom and smaller wells do not work as well as
cone-shaped wells.

2. Automatic pipette (BBL 05-687)

3. Plastic pipette tips (BBL Fibro Tip 70314, 1000 tips/box)

4. 15 cc. glass centrifuge tube

5. 1.0 ml. pipette - graduated in 1/100 ml.- one for sensitized cells

6. 0.2 ml. pipette - graduated in 1/100 ml.-one for each control
and/or patients' serum.

REAGENTS:

1. Thyroglobulin sensitized sheep cells, preserved (Burroughs
Wellcome Co., Tuckahoe, New York)

2. Control sheep cells preserved (Burroughs Wellcome Co., Tuckahoe,
New York) NOTE: Control and sensitized cells must be well shaken before
use to insure uniform suspension of cells. The control and test cells
must be from the same or matched batches. Batch cross references are
given on the bottle label. The bottle labels are color-coded; red,
control cells; black, test cells.

3. Control - Control is prepared by Quality Control. Remove
from freezer according to date. Control results are available from
Quality Control and should be confirmed before test is reported.

4. Patient's Serum - Serum is separated from clotted blood in
red top tube (no anticoagulant) by spinning in centrifuge at 2500 rpm
for 10 minutes and then pouring off to clean tube.

Procedure
    Adsorption:

1. Label 1 centrifuge tube for each control and/or patient's
serum with name and date.

66

2.   Add 0.9 ml. of well-mixed "control sheep cells" to each centrifuge tube with 1.01 ml. pipette.

3.   Using a 0.2 ml. pipette, add 0.1 ml. of control serum to control tube. Mix well.

4.   Using a 0.2 ml. pipette add 0.1 ml. patient's serum to appropriately labeled tube. Mix well.

5.   Allow to stand at room temperature for 45 minutes.

6.   Centrifuge for 5 minutes @ 2500 rpm.

7.   The supernatant, a 1/10 dilution of patient's serum free from non-specific sheep cell agglutinins, is used for the test.

TEST:

1.   To each well in a row of diluting wells, labeled 1 to 9, pipette 0.1 ml. of well-mixed "thyroglobulin sensitized sheep cells" using automatic pipette.

2.   Again using automatic pipette, add 0.1 ml. of the 1/10 dilution of adsorbed serum into well #1. Mix the serum and cells by drawing up and down in pipette three times. Transfer 0.1 ml. from well #1 into well #2. Mix. Repeat for each successive dilution up to well #9. Discard 0.1 ml. from well #9 so that 0.1 ml. of the appropriate serum dilution is left in each well.

3.   To the well labeled #10, pipette 0.1 ml. of well mixed "control sheep cells" using automatic pipette.

4.   Again using automatic pipette, add 0.1 ml. of the 1/100 dilution of adsorbed serum into well #10. Mix. Remove 0.1 ml. and discard.

5.   The final serum dilutions are as follows:

well #1	1:20	well #6	1:640
well #2	1:40	well #7	1:1280
well #3	1:80	well #8	1:2560
well #4	1:160	well #9	1:5120
well #5	1:320	well #10	neg. cont. (1:20)

6.   Cover tray with cellophane.

7.   Place on automatic rotator for 5 min. at 180 rpm.

8.   Allow to stand at room temperature overnight before reading.

READING AND REPORTING:

When the test is positive, the agglutinated cells settle as a diffuse carpet on the bottom of the well. A negative test appears as a compact button of cells on the bottom of the well. The end point is the highest dilution to give a clear positive test.

Thyroglobulin Antibody-3

The following points must be considered before reporting out any test. The control well (#10) must be negative. If agglutination is observed in control well, repeat test in the following manner. Set up wells #1-9 using "thyroglobulin sensitized cells" and serial dilution of patient's serum as is routinely done. Also set up a duplicate row of wells #1-9 using"control sheep cells" and serial dilutions of patient's serum. Titer in row using "control sheep cells" is due to non-specific sheep cell agglutinins. It must be subtracted from titer in row using "thyroglobulin sensitized cells" to obtain true titer due to thyroglobulin antibody.

If the agglutination continues through the ninth well, the test must be repeated, continuing the dilution through 18 or even 27 wells. The titer at these levels is very high and should, therefore, be rounded off before reporting.

The final serum dilutions are as follows:

well #10 - 10,240	well #15 - 327,680 = 330,000
well #11 - 20,480	well #16 - 655,360 = 650,000
well #12 - 40,960	well #17 - 1,310,720 = 1,310,000
well #13 - 81,920	well #18 - 2,621,440 = 2,620,000
well #14 - 163,840	

Thyroglobulin antibody titer - negative
Thyroglobulin antibody titer - 1:_____
                                (titers of 1:80 or over are significant)

Record results of patient's serum and control serum in Serology Day Book. Include lot no. of controls and cells in day book. Check control results with Quality Control. If results do not agree within one titer, repeat test with new control.

INTERPRETATION:

High titers, greater than 1:5000, usually indicate Hashimoto's thyroiditis or post - I131 therapy. However, positive titers may be found in cases of diffuse thyroid hyperplasia, benign and malignant thyroid neoplasia, rheumatoid arthritis and collagen disease, and a small percentage of normal population.

REFERENCES:

1. Fulthorpe, A.J., A Stable Sheep Cell Preparation for Detecting Thyroglobulin Antibodies, J. Clin. Path. 14:654, 1961.

2. Golden, M. Screening Test for Thyroid Disease as a Routine Hospital Procedure, Am. J. Clin. Path. 43:555, 1965.

January 1968 FP -1/70 -ET,CR

Figure 3-11 A thorough description of the procedure would allow a worker in another laboratory to set up and run the test without additional information. Note the references to dimensions and source of all materials; quality control procedures; pitfalls in interpretation; bibliography; date, and initials of author.

nonspecificity is not known. This is so widely practiced that to suggest the inclusion of these specifications in a procedure description may seem academic and obscure.

The Food and Drug Administration has recently been charged with the authority to evaluate and approve the quality of all biological products for use in laboratory diagnostic procedures. Ultimately this should improve the reliability of these materials and in the future may permit less attention to a definition of quality standards for biologicals in the procedure manual. At the present time the FDA lacks the resources to evaluate all biologicals before they are released on the market. Investigation usually results from a complaint which is sufficiently well documented to suggest a deficiency in the product.

When listing glassware, the dimensions of tubes and type of closure should be specified. The volume and size of pipettes used for transfer should be given. The materials list should include any control materials required.

In a description of the *performance of the procedure*, be sure to specify time. Do not use such expressions as "allow to stand," or "incubate overnight." The latter may imply anything from 12 to 24 hours. This term is often applied to the incubation of enrichment media for the isolation of enteric pathogens. It is known that 8–12 hours is the optimal period and that overgrowth of coliforms occurs in 24 hours. Similarly the incubation of bacteria in a gluconate substrate may cause metabolism of the substrate to pyruvic acid, leaving none of the intermediate product ketogluconate and resulting in a false negative reaction. Reference to centrifugation should include the revolutions per minute and the radius of the head or the gravitational force since the latter may vary with different centrifuges depending on the radius of the head. Include the use of quality control materials in the description.

The section on *technical interpretation* should follow with special attention to pitfalls that may be encountered by the inexperienced worker. Interpreting the quality control elements of the procedure should be em-

GLUCONATE OXIDATION

Place gluconate tablet in tube containing a small amount of

water. Inoculate and incubate overnight. Add a clinitest

tablet. If red precipitate forms, test is positive.

Figure 3-12 Example of inadequate description of procedure. The chemical principle is not explained. The source of materials and sizes of tubes utilized are not given. The amount of water is vague. The temperature of incubation is omitted. The time of incubation permits a range of 8–24 hours. No mention is made of quality control. There are no references and it is neither dated nor initialed.

GLUCONATE OXIDATION

PRINCIPLE:

   Gluconate salts are oxidized to Ketogluconate and thence to
pyruvic acid by certain members of the genus Pseudomonas.   An
intermediary product Ketogluconate will reduce alkaline cupric
ion with formation of a red precipitate cuprous oxide.

$$
\begin{array}{ccccc}
O = \underset{|}{CO}^- K^+ & & O = \underset{|}{CO}^- K^+ & & \underset{|}{O}^-\ K^+ \\
HCOH & & C = O & & C = O \\
HOCH & & HOCH & +Cu^{++} & HOCH \\
HCOH & \longrightarrow & HCOH & & HCOH \\
HCOH & & HCOH & +OH^- & HCOH \\
CH_2OH & & CH_2OH & & CH_2\ OH \\
& & \text{ketogluconate} & & \text{pyruvic acid (K}^+ \text{ salt)}
\end{array}
$$

Potassium gluconate

$$+Cu_2O \downarrow\downarrow$$

red precipitate

MATERIALS:

   Gluconate tablets (Key Scientific Products Co.,P.O. Box 66307,
Los Angeles 66, California)

   Clinitest tablets (Ames Div. Miles Labs, Inc.,Elkhart,Indiana)

   1 ml sterile water in 16 x 150 mm tubes with sponge closure

PROCEDURE:

   Place one gluconate tablet in tube of water aseptically.   Inoculate
heavily and incubate 18 hours at $37^{o}C$.   Test for Ketogluconate by adding
clinitest tablet.   Do not overincubate since all Ketogluconate may be
metabolized to pyruvic acid giving a false negative test.

INTERPRETATION:

   Red precipitate indicates that gluconate has been oxidized to
Ketogluconate.

REFERENCE:

   Haynes, W. C., J. of Gen. Microbiol., 5:929,1951

RCB   8/71

Figure 3-13   A proper description of a gluconate oxidation test which describes the chemical
principle; specific source of dimensions and amounts of materials; time; temperature;
warning on false negative reaction; reference; initials; and date of preparation. Quality control is covered in the surveillance schedule (see p. 198). Otherwise this should be included in
the description.

phasized. It should have been made sufficiently clear in the adminstrative section of the manual that controls must be applied according to an established schedule and that unacceptable control results require specific action. There should be no need to repeat this admonition in each procedure description. A brief section on *clinical interpretation*, including normal ranges and the significance of abnormal values, should be given. No attempt should be made to provide a comprehensive discussion suitable for either students or medical staff. It may be desirable to insert a statement supporting aspects of the test that have provoked frequent inquiries. For example, the lowest titer performed on a serologic procedure may be 1:64. Although there may be no clinical significance in lower titers, repeated inquiries by physicians can be handled more smoothly by simply stating in the description that lower titers have no clinical significance along with an appropriate reference. The *bibliography* must be given using the standard format of the Cummulative Index Medicus. Finally, the procedure must be *dated and initialed*.

Descriptions of media may follow a similar format. Because there is great variation in commercial sources of both dehydrated and prepared media it is desirable to specify a single source that is reproducible in internal laboratory quality control studies. The procedure should include a description of the preparation of the medium, even if it is obtained commercially, since this may be required in an emergency. Indicate the type of water to be used, the amounts to be weighed for typical production volumes, the method of mixing, the control of temperature during mixing, the size of glassware used in proporation to the volume prepared, and the conditions of autoclaving. Provide the length of slants and butts, the quantity or depth to be delivered in filling, and the specific size of glass- or plasticware. A separate paragraph should summarize the method of inoculation and use of the medium in the laboratory. References should be given to commercial media manuals, which are an ample source of more detailed supporting data.

QUALITY CONTROL

Techniques for introducing and administering quality control in a microbiology laboratory are discussed in Chapter 6. It is our purpose here to establish that the procedure book must contain descriptions of standards, surveillance, and control procedures. Responsibility and accountability for quality control activities is best treated in the administrative section. General standards of acceptable performance and a schedule of surveillance activities can be treated systematically in the quality control section. Therefore, in contrast to the *unique* quality control considerations given to materials and procedures in the preceding sections, a systematic approach is applicable to those *common* surveillance requirements that may be applied to all or many procedures and materials.

This section of the procedure book should begin with a list of all procedures and materials subject to surveillance. This should include a schedule for conducting surveillance and limits of variation within which performance is acceptable. A portion of this list should contain an inventory of all reagents and biological materials. The conditions of storage, expiration dates, and frequency of surveillance of adherance to these criteria should be stated. The following criteria for media can be tabulated more efficiently by a listing in the quality control section rather than with each individual description: time limits and conditions of storage for dehydrated and prepared material, pH, time and temperature of autoclaving, sterility testing, use of control cultures, labeling, and bagging. The use of positive and negative control sera with serologic tests may be outlined. When tests are performed in titer, one or more sera of known reactivity may be used. If controls are coded to reduce bias, decoding and a method for obtaining approval of control results must be described. Certain tests may be performed periodically, whether or not they are ordered on patients, and this may be outlined. An application of these principles is the surveillance schedule established in the author's laboratory (see Appendix I).

Sample forms and a description of methods of record keeping used by personnel may be provided. These should assure complete documentation of errors observed through surveillance including the date observed, to whom it was reported, corrective action taken, and whether corrective action was effective. Alternatively, personnel can determine their own methods for documenting observations if they can be made to keep systematic records which are available at any time. If a periodic report of the surveillance program is submitted to the microbiologist or director of laboratories, this procedure should be described. The ability of personnel to assume responsibility for conducting and perpetuating all elements of the system is effectively tested through a periodic summary report, such as that carried out in the author's laboratory (see Appendix). If such a report is required, it may be outlined in this section of the procedure manual.

REFERENCE DATA

This section must be bound separately from other portions of the procedure manual. The reader may argue that this is not a section of the procedure book at all, but a collection of reference data. It may consist of several notebooks or a whole filing cabinet depending on the amount of available material. There may be no more than one copy or set maintained by the microbiologist, and it may consist primarily of reprints, tables, and other information used for working out problems encountered with unusual specimens and isolates. There would be little purpose in reproducing this material for personnel who are issued copies of basic sections of the manual. This greatly reduces the volume of the material to be reproduced and facilitates additions, deletions, and revisions of reference material. It should be monitored once a year to eliminate obsolete and redundant data.

## CHAPTER 4

Information Systems

WHAT PRIORITY FOR COMMUNICATION?

Chapter 1 discussed the contemporary social challenge to achieve a more efficient and economical application of our technical capabilities to human problems. Those responsible for directing microbiology laboratories have often placed a higher priority on technology than on communication.

Time allows progressive academic refinement of the microbiologic report, but bears an inverse relation to the value of the report for patient care. The problem would be minimized if observations could be reported at each progressive step of evaluation. Unfortunately most laboratories are limited to one preliminary report; indeed many are unable to manage more than one final report. Limited space often results in terse handwritten phrasing which is misinterpreted. Independent laboratories, unlike hospital laboratories, have no captive market. Competition has focused attention on providing the physician-consumer with the most attractive product. Although there is evidence of substandard practice in some of these laboratories, most provide better service without compromising quality. A little competition would bring about some rapid improvements in the reporting practices of hospital laboratories.

The processing of all laboratory information by automatic data systems will probably be universal within a few years. Much additional development and experience is required to increase economy and efficiency and thus achieve a more impressive cost-benefit ratio. In the meantime, most laboratories are dependent on various forms that minimize handwritten information and transcription. An intermediate step toward automatic data processing is a cumulative reporting system utilizing electrostatic copies.

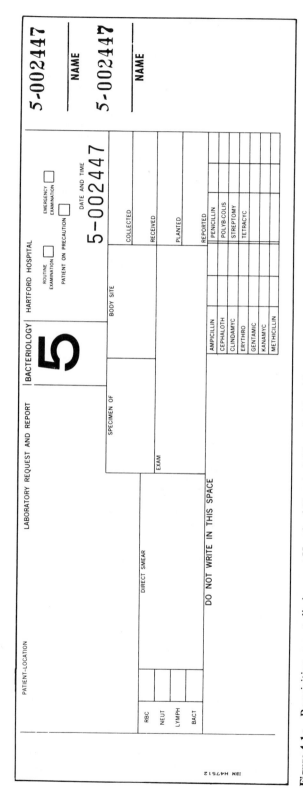

Figure 4-1a Requisition-report slip in use at Hartford Hospital. Note the identification stickers for use on the specimen.

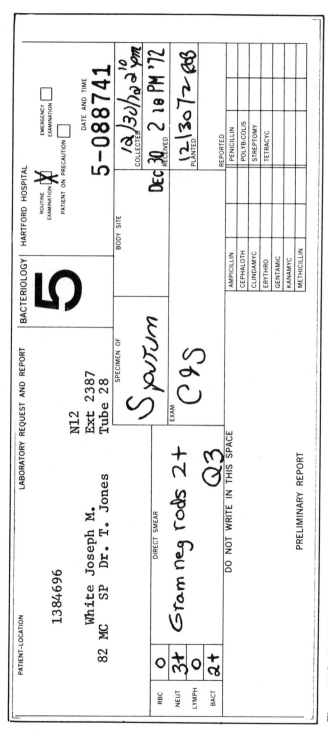

Figure 4-1b Preliminary report copy.

Figure 4-1c Final report copy. These are "shingled" into the medical record leaving the lower portion of the slip visible. Other information is observed by turning up the overlying slip. Note the documentation of date and time collected and received; and date planted and reported. The final report was rendered after 5 days. A second preliminary report should have been provided after 48 hours giving the species isolated before confirmatory antimicrobial susceptibility tests were performed. The preliminary report slip had been used to report Gram stain results. Personnel were reluctant to fill out an entire new slip for this purpose. Progressive updating of reports is easier with electrostatic cumulative copy system. Computerized reporting enables an even more convenient revision of sequential preliminary report. Now a new cumulative electrostatic copy system is being used to render preliminary and final reports. The requisition-report slip is being used only as a requisition and work card.

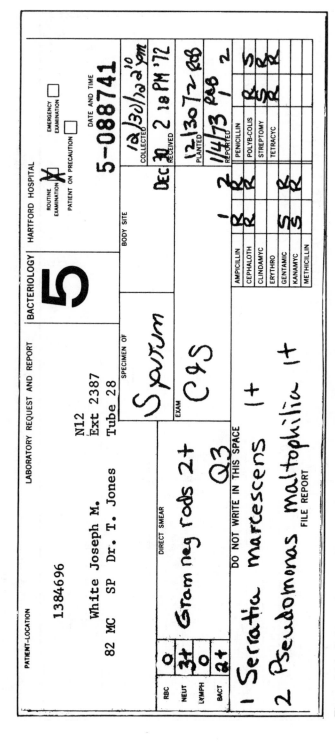

Figure 4-1d Laboratory copy (file report). The front side provides a carbon copy of the report.

1 2

| + – POSITIVE | D – DELAYED | F – FERMENTATIVE | AG – ACID GAS |
| 0 – NEGATIVE | OX – OXIDATIVE | A – ACID | ALK. – ALKALINE |

Handwritten notes:

12/31 1) lg G-rod 1+
2) Sm G-rod → Mœ isol.

1/1 ?. maybe sens mixed → repeat

1/2 18° broth

1/3 tube gentamicin

1/4 Gent. (R)

TSI SLANT	K K	IND.		TSN	SALMON-ELLA	POLY d vi
TSI BUTT	A	O	M.R.		INOS.		A B C₁ C₂ D E F G H I
H₂S	+		V.P.		MAL.	SHIGELLA A B C D
ORN.	+		NIT.	+		POLY E. COLI A B C
MOT.	+		MAC.			HEMOPHILUS A B
LYS.			GEL.		√ OF GLUC.	ARIZONA POLY	O H
ONPG	%		GLUC. OX.		√ OF MALT	ALK-DISPAR O
UREA WET PREP	+		PSEUDO		OF LACT	BETH-BAL. POLY
PAD					OF SUC	FLUORES. ANTIB.
DNASE	+		CAT.		OF XYL	NORMAL FLORA
ARAB.	O		COAG.		CTA GLUC	MIXED FLORA
OXID.	O		PSE		CTA MALT	C.C. GREATER THAN 10⁵
PIG.			6.5 SALT		CTA SUC	C.C. 10⁴-10⁵
			BILE		CTA LACT	C.C. LESS THAN 10⁴

Figure 4-1e Reverse of laboratory copy (file report). This is used as a worksheet for recording all observations. The tabular arrangement facilitates a review of the work by a supervisor.

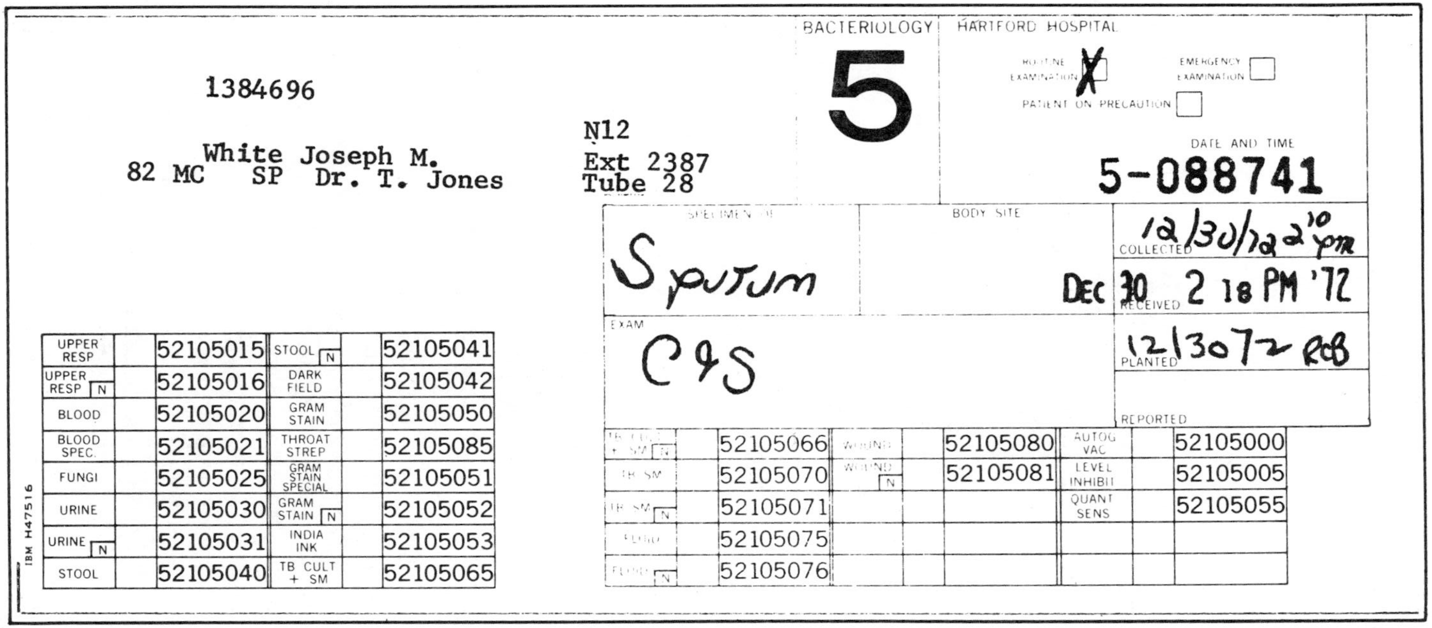

BACTERIOLOGY | HARTFORD HOSPITAL

5

ROUTINE EXAMINATION [X] EMERGENCY EXAMINATION [ ]
PATIENT ON PRECAUTION [ ]

1384696

82 MC White Joseph M. SP Dr. T. Jones

N12
Ext 2387
Tube 28

DATE AND TIME
5-088741

SPECIMEN OF: Sputum
BODY SITE
EXAM: C&S

COLLECTED 12/30/72 2[10] pm
RECEIVED DEC 30 2 18 PM '72
PLANTED 12/30/72 RCB
REPORTED

UPPER RESP		52105015	STOOL N	52105041
UPPER RESP N		52105016	DARK FIELD	52105042
BLOOD		52105020	GRAM STAIN	52105050
BLOOD SPEC.		52105021	THROAT STREP	52105085
FUNGI		52105025	GRAM STAIN SPECIAL	52105051
URINE		52105030	GRAM STAIN N	52105052
URINE N		52105031	INDIA INK	52105053
STOOL		52105040	TB CULT + SM	52105065

TB CULT + SM N		52105066	WOUND		52105080	AUTOG VAC		52105000
TB SM		52105070	WOUND N		52105081	LEVEL INHIBIT		52105005
TB SM N		52105071				QUANT SENS		52105055
FLUID		52105075						
FLUID N		52105076						

IBM H47516

Figure 4-1*f* Charge card. Requisition report slip is now used only as a requisition. Reports are provided through electrostatic cumulative copy system. (See Figure 4-5). Preliminary and final report forms shown (*b*) and (*c*) are no longer used. Laboratory copy (*d*, *e*) and charge card (*f*) continue in use.

The author's laboratory has evolved from the use of "IBM type" requisition-report slips to such a cumulative reporting system. In addition certain specific automatic data systems applications have been developed in our laboratory.

REPORT FORMS

The requisition and report form used for bacteriology is illustrated in Figure 4-1. Formerly, this was used by us for all bacteriology reporting. The form is now used only for its function as a requisition and work card because bacteriology reports are rendered by the electrostatic copy system using the cumulative reports described in the following pages. Reports continue to be made on these forms for specimens submitted for isolation of fungi and mycobacteria.

The following description for using these slips refers to their application prior to the introduction of the electrostatic cumulative copy system. Information of interest to the physician is located on the lower portion, allowing the slips to be entered into the chart in a "shingled" fashion. Similar slips are used for other procedures that may be performed in the microbiology laboratory, such as parasitology, clinical microscopy, and immunology. Space is provided for entry of the date and time of collection, arrival at the laboratory, planting, and reporting. The original or front copy of the slip becomes the final report. A second page is marked "preliminary report" and may be torn out and sent to the chart prior to the final report.

The increasing demand for preliminary reporting is being felt in most laboratories. We know of no laboratory that has attempted to render preliminary reports on all bacteriologic specimens with a standard manual reporting system because of the substantial clerical burden that would result.

The third page of our requisition-report slip is the laboratory copy. Space is provided for writing observations made on cultures and notes regarding transfers. On the reverse side there is a section for recording the results of all biochemical and serologic observations that lead to identification. Information recorded on preliminary and final report portions of the slip is transmitted by carbon to the laboratory copy. The laboratory file copies are reviewed by the supervisor who insures that all information is properly recorded and that the specified number of criteria support identification. The final page of the form is the charge card. This is removed as soon as the specimen arrives in the laboratory. Credit cards are prepared when tests are not performed.

Our slips have attached gummed numbered labels which are removed for identifying specimens. Systems that provide multiple adhesive labels from the patient's wrist band, providing greater assurance of patient identification, are now available. Some message should be placed on these report slips when specimens are received without identification on the container. We use a stamp that states "Identification by slip—container not labeled." We have been advised that this may absolve the laboratory of liability for performing tests on unlabeled specimens. Specimens that are received with no label on either the requisition slip or the container are discarded.

Increasing emphasis should be placed on the time of collection and receipt in the laboratory. This allows the development of specific criteria for accepting specimens that have not been excessively delayed with resulting deterioration. Also it is valuable for arbitrating disputes over delays that allegedly have occurred in the laboratory.

Terminology used in reports should be well standardized and legible. This may be facilitated by the use of rubber stamps. Their use, as well as the application of standard handwritten terminology, should be defined in the procedure manual as described in Chapter 3. Special messages are common on bacteriology reports. It is especially important that these be highly standardized to avoid misinterpretation. It is important that the medical and nursing staff be fully apprised of the rationale behind reports indicating the unacceptability of specimens since these are often provocative. Methods of notifying personnel of these policies were reviewed in the previous chapter and a discussion of their clinical justification appeared in Chapter 2. Stamps used to convey these messages in the author's laboratory are illustrated in Figure 4-2. Figure 4-3 lists specimens which were inferior for a variety of reasons, or required additional information, resulting in limited or no processing and a request for repeat collection or a consultation. A communication written to justify and clarify our policy of requesting consultations or repeat collections on inferior specimens is shown in Figure 4-4.

RAPID REPORTING

Some microbiologists are experiencing either telephone calls or visits to the laboratory by house staff with lists of patients from whom specimens have been submitted on the previous day. Either preliminary reports must be rendered on specimens of major interest or disorganization and delay in reporting will result from an increase in such inquiries. We have established a rule that some report will be rendered within 48 hours on specimens submitted for culture, and on the same day when direct examinations are requested. There is nothing unusual about this standard but it is surprising how often 4 or 5 days elapse while the laboratory worker loses sight of the length of time he has been studying the specimen (see Figure 1-2). The simple observation that a culture contains growth and is not sterile may not impress laboratory workers preoccupied with speciation and sensitivity testing of the isolate. Ironically, rapid reporting of the presence or absence of growth may have a greater impact on diagnosis and treatment than more detailed information which is reported later.

To be used on any specimen except CSF, blood and feces when more than one specimen is submitted in one day.

SEE RESULTS REPORTED ON DUPLICATE SPECIMEN RECEIVED

Used when additional information is required prior to processing specimen or when request is of doubtful clinical value (culture of mouth, anaerobic culture of expectorated sputum, etc.)

CONSULTATION REQUIRED FOR PERFORMANCE OF TEST

Used to report specimens requesting N. gonorrhoeae when none was isolated.

NO NEISSERIA GONORRHOEAE ISOLATED

Used to report feces cultures when no pathogens are isolated.

FECES CULTURE NEGATIVE FOR STAPHYLOCOCCI,
SALMONELLA, AND SHIGELLA

Used to report feces cultures on children under 2 years of age when no entero-pathogenic E. coli is isolated.

CULTURE NEGATIVE FOR ENTEROPATHOGENIC
E. COLI GROUPS A, B AND C

Used to report sterile blood cultures.

CULTURE STERILE AFTER 2 WEEKS INCUBATION

Used to report requests for anaerobic culture.

NO ANAEROBES ISOLATED AFTER _____ DAYS

Used to report any other sterile culture except blood, urine and anaerobic cultures.

CULTURE STERILE AFTER _____ DAYS INCUBATION

Used as stated by stamp

IDENTIFICATION BY SLIP.   CONTAINER NOT LABELED

Used on specimens which show the same bacterial isolates as the previous day on the same type of specimen.

NO SIGNIFICANT CHANGE FROM PREVIOUS SPECIMEN

Used in reporting colony counts on all urine cultures.

> 100,000 colonies/cc

10,000 - 100,000 colonies/cc

< 10,000 colonies/cc

Used to report sterile clean catch and indwelling catheter urine cultures.

Sterile or < 1,000 bacteria/mL.

For reporting of improperly submitted specimens.

PLEASE SUBMIT ANOTHER SPECIMEN
RECEIVED AFTER PROLONGED DELAY ☐ WRONG CONTAINER ☐
INADEQUATE SPECIMEN ☐ CONTAMINATION ☐ CLOTTED ☐

Used on specimens submitted from lower respiratory tract when the number of potential pathogens exceeds the quality of the specimen.

Mixed culture of: Staph aur ☐ Staph ep ☐ Strep ☐ D pneumo ☐ Yeast ☐
Corynbac ☐ E coli ☐ Klebs/Ent ☐ Proteus ☐ Non ferm Gram·neg rods ☐

Evidence of oropharyngeal contamination-please repeat.

Specimens collected from tracheostomies when the number of potential pathogens exceeds the quality of the specimen.

Mixed culture of: Staph aur ☐ Staph ep ☐ Strep ☐ D pneumo ☐ Yeast ☐
Corynbac ☐ E coli ☐ Klebs/Ent ☐ Proteus ☐ Non ferm Gram neg rods ☐

Evidence of stomal area contamination-please repeat.

Used on clean catch and indwelling catheter urine specimens when 3 or more organisms are isolated.

Mixed culture of: Staph aur ☐ Staph ep ☐ Strep ☐ D pneumo ☐ Yeast ☐
Corynbac ☐ E coli ☐ Klebs/Ent ☐ Proteus ☐ Non ferm Gram neg rods ☐

Probable contamination-please repeat.

To be used on any type of specimen to report beta hemolytic streptococcus not Group A.

BETA-HEMOLYTIC STREP NOT GROUP A

Used to report Group A strep isolated from any type of specimen.

BETA-HEMOLYTIC STREP GROUP A

Used to report throat cultures when no beta hemolytic strep is isolated.

NO BETA HEMOLYTIC STREP ISOLATED

Figure 4-2   Stamps for frequently used statements on reports.

"Consultation required for performance of test"		
Urine, fungus	11	
Blood, fungus	4	
Feces, fungus	1	
Resp. tract, fungus, anaerobes	6	
Mouth	5	
Vomitus	2	
Throat (fungi)	1	
Foley tips	21	
		51
		—
"Please submit another specimen . . .		
Delay"		
Urine		
Time not given	208	
>4 hours	36	
received after 10 p.m.	53	
Stools		
Date not given	1	
received after 10 p.m.	5	
Fluids or wounds		
Time not given	5	
>6 hours	4	
received after 10 p.m.	38	
Sputum		
Time not given	7	
>6 hours	19	
received after 10 p.m.	33	
		409
		—
"Wrong container"		
Urines	6	
Fluids or wounds	3	
Sputum	1	
		10
		—

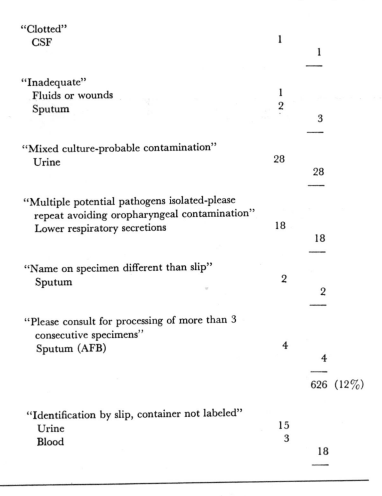

"Clotted"
CSF   1
                                                                    1
                                                                   —

"Inadequate"
Fluids or wounds   1
Sputum   2
                                                                    3
                                                                   —

"Mixed culture-probable contamination"
Urine   28
                                                                   28
                                                                   —

"Multiple potential pathogens isolated-please
  repeat avoiding oropharyngeal contamination"
Lower respiratory secretions   18
                                                                   18
                                                                   —

"Name on specimen different than slip"
Sputum   2
                                                                    2
                                                                   —

"Please consult for processing of more than 3
  consecutive specimens"
Sputum (AFB)   4
                                                                    4
                                                                   —
                                                            626 (12%)

"Identification by slip, container not labeled"
Urine   15
Blood   3
                                                                   18
                                                                   —

Figure 4-3 Of 5200 specimens received in August 1972 in the author's laboratory, 626 (12%) required additional information for processing, were received after prolonged delay or in incorrect containers, or were reported as mixed cultures without speciation. Specimens were refrigerated for 72 hours pending a call from the physician and repeat collection was requested. Only rare requests were received to process inferior specimens. Most consultations that were requested did not occur. See our letter to the medical staff concerning this problem (Figure 4-4).

Providing information that is only 80% secure in 12 hours is of more clinical value than information that is 98% secure in 48 hours. Microbiologists tend to delay reporting partly because of academic or professional anxiety about giving insecure information, but perhaps chiefly because preliminary statements require a second final confirmation, a clerical burden and cost that most laboratories have not been able to sustain. Some laboratories provide telephone reports only when "Stat" or emergency examinations have been requested. Workers often overlook the fact that their written reports must subsequently be collated by clerical

H A R T F O R D   H O S P I T A L

H A R T F O R D ,   C O N N E C T I C U T   0 6 1 1 5

Dear Doctor:

The number of specimens submitted to the Microbiology Division of the Department of Pathology have continued to increase. Simultaneously our work has grown in complexity through: an improved reporting system; greater accuracy in isolation and identification; quality control; new tests.

The hospital administration, in response to pressure from public agencies and third party payers, has been exerting tight control over increases in personnel. No automation is available to improve efficiency in Microbiology. The public is telling us that they will not continue to pay for rising hospital costs, which have grown 126% in 5 years. A significant portion of this are laboratory costs which have soared 229% over the same period.

Only two alternatives are open to us. Either we reduce quality and accommodate the increase; or we monitor and control the quality of the material which we accept. We believe that the quality of clinical microbiology performed here is above average and have heard no claim that it is excessive or irrelevant. The time may come when the public will refuse to pay for above average health services. In the meantime we are pursuing the second alternative.

During one month the following suboptimal specimens were submitted to us. Repeats were requested. All specimens were saved for 72 hours pending a consultation with the physician should processing be clinically and microbiologically preferable to recollection.

Urines, no time of collection	208
Urines, more than 4 hour delay	36
Received after 10 pm (no call received)	149
Insufficient information, consultation requested	51
Received on day after collection; wrong container; clotted; insufficient; contaminated	95
Total	539

This represents: a saving of about $4,300.00 in charges each month; a reduction in the number of personnel required to operate this division from 28 to 25; elimination of misleading information resulting from deterioration and contamination of specimens.

We are hearing indirect and vague complaints that we are arbitrarily restricting service and throwing out specimens. Most physicians assume that a request for consultation or repeat collection indicates that the specimen has been discarded. Processing of inferior specimens requires a discussion with the physician of the relative merits of collecting another. We cannot call on each of the five hundred odd occasions that this occurs each month. Instead we are trying to issue written reports promptly. Occasionally our personnel mishandle specimens. If you believe that this has occurred or wish to discuss any problem regarding collection and processing of specimens or interpretation of reports, please call me at my office (Ext. 2206) or at home (658-5868).

Sincerely yours,

Raymond C. Bartlett, M.D.
Division of Microbiology
Department of Pathology

RCB:jg

Figure 4-4   Letter sent to medical staff summarizing the data shown in Figure 4-3.

personnel and delivered through a tube system, by messenger, or through the mail. There is usually a delay of at least half a day between the time the final report is written and appears on the patient's chart. Mailed reports are delayed even longer.

It is difficult to establish priorities for the types of information that should be reported by telephone. A high priority should be placed on telephone or rapid preliminary reporting of information that affects the immediate treatment of life threatening conditions or isolation of patients. Examples are positive smears or cultures of blood and spinal fluid, or isolation of *Salmonella, Shigella*, and *Enteropathogenic Escherichia coli*. Pressure applied by clinicians may also affect priorities. For example, children seen for acute pharyngitis in the Emergency and Outpatient Departments of Hartford Hospital are cultured and instructed on treatment by telephone on the following day. This results in a demand for all of the previous day's throat culture results, complete with grouping of streptococci, by noon on the day after they are received by the laboratory. Our employee and student health clinics have requested results early each day to allow personnel without serious or hazardous infections to return to work or classes.

At the Massachusetts General Hospital the bacteriology laboratory began receiving early morning calls to determine whether there was bacterial growth in urine or blood cultures that had been submitted on the previous day. This practice was generated by an aggressive house staff which found it clinically useful to indicate on morning rounds whether there was any growth in such specimens. This was a major factor in causing Dr. Lawrence Kunz, director of that laboratory, to develop a computerized information system. One microbiology laboratory was so besieged with morning telephone calls for results that a rule was established permitting no telephone inquiries before 10 a.m.

Instantaneous analysis and immediate reporting of results on all microbiologic specimens would be a valuable adjunct to rapid diagnosis and treatment. We are limited in rendering such a service by technology, manual processing of information, and the need to batch work for maximum efficiency. The laboratory director may individualize processing and reporting with as many specimens as can be accommodated by the number of technical and clerical personnel that the hospital administration will provide. At the same time the laboratory director should investigate the internal priorities of the microbiology laboratory, where personnel time may be allocated to activities less relevant to improved patient care.

Supplementary statements help to bring about more rapid final reporting. It may be a question of semantics whether one is rendering a preliminary and final report, or a final and supplementary report. We have observed instances in which additional information was expected on isolates submitted to reference laboratories prior to a final report. For example, a report of "*Pseudomonas sp.* isolated" would be more useful than the preliminary report stating "Gram negative rods isolated." A supplementary report can be issued when reference laboratory results assist in establishing precise speciation. The microbiologist must recognize that supplements based on several weeks of additional work may not come to the attention of the physician if the patient has been discharged. The final identification of a mycobacterium as *Mycobacterium intracellulare* may modify the physician's approach to the case if he had received a preliminary report that a *Mycobacterium sp.* had been isolated. The same obviously is true of an elevated fungus serology titer received from a reference laboratory and placed directly in the patient's medical record after discharge.

CUMULATIVE REPORTING SYSTEM

Those who are not medically initiated and inured to the practice of shuffling through a medical record in search of laboratory data are appalled by its chaos. Reports are shingled one after another, often without regard to date, type of specimen, or test. An entire 8 ½ × 11 sheet often contains only two or three test results. Many an intern has spent an hour in the middle of the night preparing a chart that would finally make it possible to interpret a series of chemical, hematologic, and microbiologic reports. House officers today demand that this be done by clerks and computers. Varying amounts of pressure is being applied to laboratories by the medical staff to provide such reporting systems. This is not accomplished without a moderate reorganization of laboratory activity and the addition of clerical staff. Once again the hospital administration must reconcile the cost with the value of the service. The following system was developed in the Microbiology Division at Hartford Hospital.

Cumulative reporting was applied only to bacteriology. Mycology and mycobacteriology are still reported on the conventional report slip. A cumulative report form that was developed appears in Figure 4-5. Reorganization of technologists' activities was required. Previously each technologist spent 1 week on a bench performing urine cultures and then moved on to another bench processing respiratory specimens. This system requires that all specimens received on any given patient be processed at the same bench. Specimens are divided alphabetically into eight different groups, A–C, D–G, and so forth. The requisition report slip previously described continues to be used by nursing personnel to establish identification, type of specimen, examination requested, and date and time of collection and receipt in the laboratory. The laboratory copy of this slip is used to document planting and observations made on cultures, transfers, and biochemical and serologic tests for identification.

At the time of planting the technologist looks in a loose-leaf notebook kept on her bench for a cumulative report card showing the patient's name and history number. If none is found, she assumes that this is the first bacteriologic specimen received on that patient and a new card is prepared and inserted in the book. Results of Gram stain, culture, and susceptibility testing are recorded on the cumulative card. All cards on which new information has been written are submitted to a clerk for copying at noon each day. The machine that is used automatically enters the date on the copy.

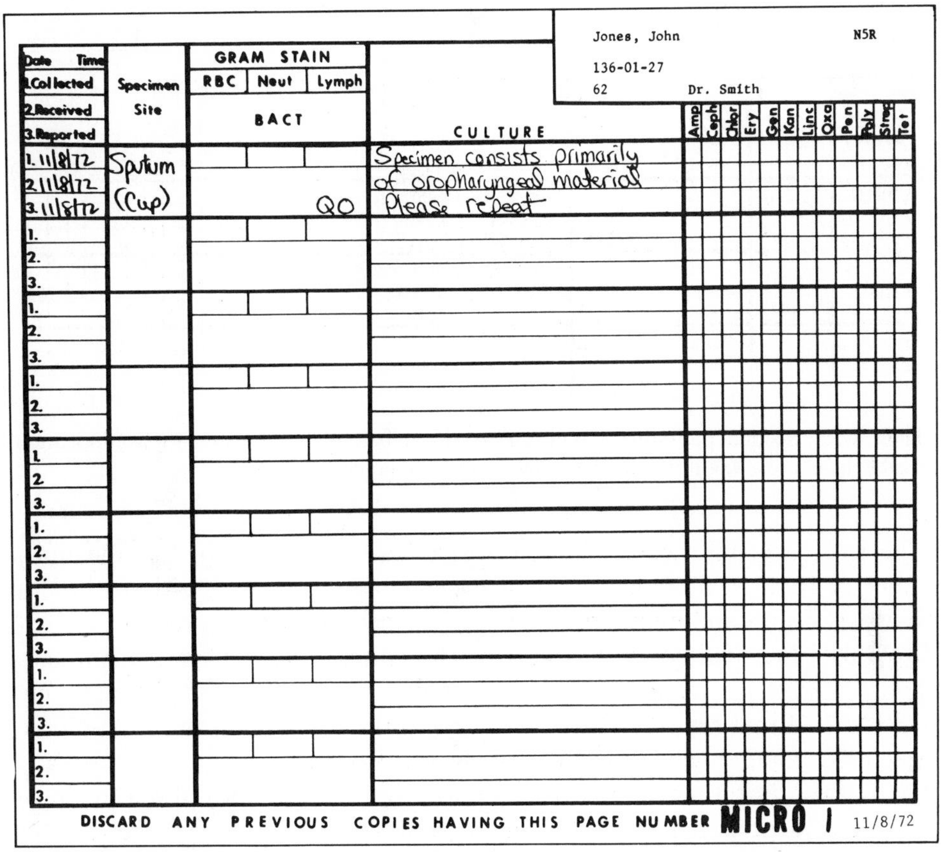

GRAM STAIN — Figure 4-5a

Date Time 1.Collected 2.Received 3.Reported	Specimen Site	RBC	Neut	Lymph BACT	CULTURE	Amp Ceph Chlor Ery Gen Kan Linc Oxa Pen Poly Strep Tet
1.11/8/72 2.11/8/72 3.11/8/72	Sputum (Cup)			QO	Specimen consists primarily of oropharyngeal material Please repeat	

Jones, John N5R
136-01-27
62 Dr. Smith

DISCARD ANY PREVIOUS COPIES HAVING THIS PAGE NUMBER **MICRO I** 11/8/72

Figure 4-5a Electrostatic copy of card kept at the laboratory bench for sequential entry of data on specimens. This record indicates poor quality sputum specimen (Q-O, see p. 58 for explanation) and requests repeat. The date of preparation is entered automatically by the electrostatic copy machine in the lower right hand corner.

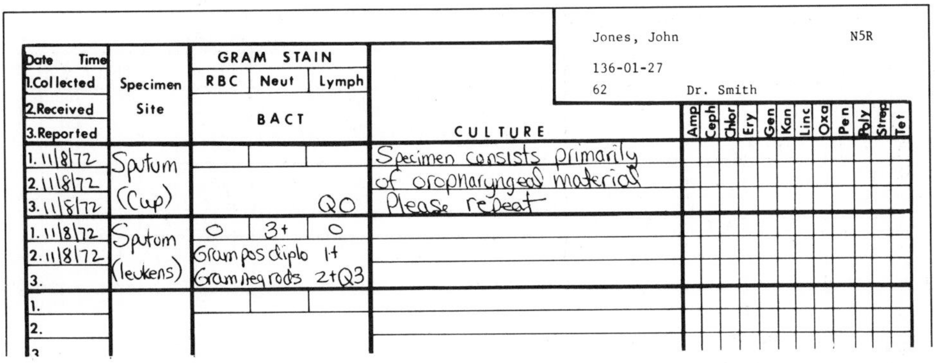

GRAM STAIN — Figure 4-5b

Date Time 1.Collected 2.Received 3.Reported	Specimen Site	RBC	Neut	Lymph BACT	CULTURE	Amp Ceph Chlor Ery Gen Kan Linc Oxa Pen Poly Strep Tet
1.11/8/72 2.11/8/72 3.11/8/72	Sputum (Cup)			QO	Specimen consists primarily of oropharyngeal material Please repeat	
1.11/8/72 2.11/8/72 3.	Sputum (leukens)	O Gram pos diplo	3+	O 1+ Gram neg rods 2+ Q3		

Jones, John N5R
136-01-27
62 Dr. Smith

Figure 4-5b A repeat specimen is received, logged in, and a preliminary report giving the gram stain results is rendered on the same day (Q-3 indicates that the specimen is of good quality).

Figure 4-5c Second preliminary report is rendered based on the extent of identification possible from gross examination and rapid testing of colonies.

Patient care unit secretaries are instructed to discard all but the most recent copy of each report. When one cumulative report card is filled, a second is begun and numbered Page 2. It is necessary to prevent accidental disposal of the final copy of Page 1 by the unit secretary when the first facsimile of Page 2 is received. This is accomplished by labeling the last copy of Page 1 "Final report." These are sent to the floors by a pneumatic tube system. Computer generated lists of discharged patients are received each day by the laboratory. Cards from these patients are removed and a single final copy is prepared and retained by the laboratory. The original master cumulative report is sent to Medical Records. The medical records department removes the laboratory duplicate that was used during hospitalization, discards it, and replaces it with the original. This assures that the original laboratory record is permanently a part of the patient's medical record.

Figure 4-5d The final report provides species and results of antimicrobial susceptibility testing. Correcting the preliminary species identification shown in the previous report is accomplished by placing a strip of blank lined tape over the area on the master card. Updated information is written in this area.

Date / Time	Specimen Site	GRAM STAIN			CULTURE	Amp	Ceph	Chlor	Ery	Gen	Kan	Linc	Oxa	Pen	Poly	Strep	Tet
1. Collected / 2. Received / 3. Reported		RBC	Neut	Lymph / BACT													
1. 11/8/72 / 2. 11/8/72 / 3. 11/8/72	Sputum (Cup)			QO	Specimen consists primarily of oropharyngeal material Please repeat												
1. 11/8/72 / 2. 11/8/72 / 3. 11/10/72	Sputum (leukens)	O / Gram pos diplo 1+	3+ / Gram neg rods 2+Q3	O	Diplococcus pneumoniae 2+ Klebsiella pneumoniae 2+	R	S			S	S				S	S	S
1. 11/10/72 / 2. 11/10/72 / 3.	Blood																
1. 11/10/72 / 2. 11/10/72 / 3.	Blood																
1. 11/10/72 / 2. 11/10/72 / 3.	Blood																
1. 11/11/72 7AM / 2. 11/11/72 1PM / 3. 11/11/72	Urine				PLEASE SUBMIT ANOTHER SPECIMEN RECEIVED AFTER PROLONGED DELAY ☒ WRONG CONTAINER ☐ INADEQUATE SPECIMEN ☐ CONTAMINATION ☐ CLOTTED ☒												
1. 11/11/72 4PM / 2. 11/11/72 5PM / 3. 11/12/72	Urine				MIXED CULTURE, PROBABLE CONTAMINATION, PLEASE REPEAT												
1. 11/12/72 8AM / 2. 11/12/72 9AM / 3. 11/14/72	Urine				Escherichia coli >100,000/ml	S	S			S	S				S	S	S
1. 11/13/72 / 2. 11/13/72 / 3. 11/14/72	leg ulcer	O / Gram pos and neg rods and cocci 4+	occ	occ	Mixed cutaneous and intestinal flora. Represents mixed infection or superficial contamination Esb												

Patient header: Jones, John   N5R   136-01-27   62   Dr. Smith

DISCARD   ANY   PREVIOUS   COPIES   HAVING   THIS   PAGE   NUMBER   **MICRO 1**   11/14/72

Figure 4-5*e*   A copy of the completed card. A reminder at the base of the card to discard previous copies prevents daily accumulation of older copies of this page in the medical record. Because of the risk that this copy of Page 1 may be discarded by the ward clerk when the first copy of Page 2 is received, this report is prominently stamped "Do Not Discard." Note that final reports have not been entered on blood cultures. After 2 weeks incubation these are recorded as sterile on the original. Another copy representing the final report of Page 1 is sent to the medical record.

When this system was introduced transient confusion and dissatisfaction among workers resulted from the reorganization of activities and added clerical work. In time the clinical and laboratory value of the report bacame apparent to laboratory personnel who would not now consider returning to the older system. Division of work among personnel by patients grouped alphabetically was required. The more efficient and common practice in large laboratories of dividing work among personnel by type of specimen results in a lack of familiarity with the bacteriologic problems of individual patients. For example, two technologists may separately work up the same atypical Gram negative rod on the same patient, one from a urine specimen and the other from a blood culture. The cumulative report instantly makes apparent all work previously performed on the patient. Although this may bias the technologist, we believe that this risk is outweighed by the advantages which include: recognition that duplicate specimens have been received, misindentification that may have occurred if a different but related species to that reported on a previous day is about to be recorded, and reduction of complete speciation and antimicrobial susceptibility testing on specimens received on sequential days. These policies were discussed in Chapter 2. They could not have been implemented without a cumulative recording and reporting system.

AUTOMATIC INFORMATION SYSTEMS

It is not difficult to *speculate* on the potential advantages of automatic processing of microbiologic information. Unfortunately there has been limited experience with applying this technique. This is due to the higher priority established for processing clinical chemistry data because of its greater volume, ease of manipulating numerical results, and opportunity for direct interfacing of instruments. This has provided a substantial opportunity to reduce costs while simultaneously improving the speed of delivery, organization, and legibility of reports. Those with experience in preliminary efforts at data systems applications in microbiology acknowledge that there may be no saving. It will probably be more costly to apply *at least* for the first few years. Justification depends on a comparison of the cost-benefit ratio with innumerable other improvements that are constantly being proposed to advance patient care. Someone must amass enough information and judgment to decide which of these proposals will be introduced without driving hospital costs beyond the limits of public acceptance.

With rare exception, commercially available systems provide assessioning and reporting for microbiology based on the pattern established for clinical chemistry data. Although this is a good place to begin, these systems fail to apply the computer to many of the unique features of clinical microbiology from which major improvements in patient care could be derived.

A system developed by the Laboratory for Computer Science, in cooperation with Lawrence J. Kunz, Ph.D., Chief of the Bacteriology Laboratory at the Massachusetts General Hospital, demonstrates many of the unique features that can be applied in bacteriology. This system also takes into account many individual needs of the institution for which it was designed. Although it allowed a reduction in laboratory clerical staff and greatly improved the efficiency of technologists, amortization of the cost for development and maintenance probably exceeded manpower savings. It is quite apparent that if one starts from scratch with program development and attempts to meet as many unique needs as this system does, there would be no way to justify the cost if it were financed through the usual sources of income available to support laboratory services.

Tapes and documentation are available at nominal cost from the Laboratory of Computer Science at the Massachusetts General Hospital for use by

```
04/10/72     12N MGH              WHITE, THOMAS B    GR3AS    76-60-72


                 ---SPUTUM

04/08 SPUTUM      SN:5184
      SMEAR..ABUNDANT GRAM POSITIVE COCCI IN PAIRS, CHAINS AND
         ..CLUSTERS. ABUNDANT SMALL GRAM POSITIVE AND GRAM
         ..NEGATIVE RODS, MODERATE GRAM NEGATIVE DIPLOCOCCI.
         ..ABUNDANT CELLS ? OF TYPE
      CULTURE:  PEND


04/08 SPUTUM      SN:5277
      SMEAR..READ BY DOCTOR
      CULTURE:  PEND

04/09 SPUTUM      SN:5534     PEND
```

Figure 4-6a Series of cumulative and updated reports generated by a computerized information system in the bacteriology laboratory at Massachusetts General Hospital. Note the first entry of sputum on 4/9 (SN:5534) as pending. This notifies the floor at the noon report that it has been received but no results are available. Note the free entry of observations on Gram stain of previous sputum specimen SN:5184.

```
04/10/72     4PM MGH              WHITE, THOMAS B    GR3AS    76:60-72




                 ----SPUTUM

04/08 SPUTUM      SN:5184
      SMEAR..ABUNDANT GRAM POSITIVE COCCI IN PAIRS, CHAINS AND
         ..CLUSTERS,ABUNDANT SMALL GRAM POSITIVE AND GRAM
         ..NEGATIVE RODS, MODERATE GRAM NEGATIVE DIPLOCOCCI.
         ..ABUNDANT CELLS ? OF TYPE
      CULTURE:
      ABUNDANT STAPH AUREUS
      VERY SCANT NORMAL THROAT FLORA PRESENT


04/08 SPUTUM      SN:5277
      SMEAR..READ BY DOCTOR
      CULTURE:
      ABUNDANT STAPH AUREUS
      NORMAL THROAT THROAT ABSENT


04/09 SPUTUM      SN:5534
      VERY RARE PROTEUS SPECIES..OVERGROWING CULTURE
      ABUNDANT GRAM NEGATIVE RODS
      ? OF ABUNDANT STAPH SPECIES
```

Figure 4-6b The 4 p.m. report on the same day indicates general observations made on the culture.

```
04/11/72    12N MGH                    WHITE, THOMAS B    GR3AS    76-60-72


                    ----SPUTUM

04/08  SPUTUM    SN:5184
       SMEAR..ABUNDANT GRAM POSITIVE COCCI IN PAIRS,CHAINS AND
             ..CLUSTERS.ABUNDANT SMALL GRAM POSITIVE AND GRAM
             ..NEGATIVE RODS,MODERATE GRAM NEGATIVE DIPLOCOCCI
             ..ABUNDANT CELLS ? OF TYPE
       CULTURE:
       ABUNDANT STAPH AUREUS
          PEN R    METH S    ERYTH S    CEPH S    TETRA S
          CHLOR S
       VERY SCANT NORMAL THROAT FLORA PRESENT

04/08  SPUTUM    SN:5277
       SMEAR..READ BY DOCTOR
       CULTURE:
       ABUNDANT STAPH AUREUS
       NORMAL THROAT FLORA ABSENT

04/09  SPUTUM    SN:5534
       VERY RARE PROTEUS SPECIES..OVERGROWING CULTURE
       ABUNDANT GRAM NEGATIVE RODS
          CEPH R    TETRA S    CHLOR I    AMP S    STREP S
          KANA S    GENTA S    COLI S
       ? OF ABUNDANT STAPH SPECIES
```

Figure 4-6c   Results of susceptibility testing are reported the next day at noon.

```
04/11/72    4 PM MGH                    WHITE, THOMAS B    GR3AS    76-60-72



                    ----SPUTUM

04/08  SPUTUM    SN:5184
####   FINAL REPORT:
       SMEAR..ABUNDANT GRAM POSITIVE COCCI IN PAIRS,CHAINS AND
             ..CLUSTERS.ABUNDANT SMALL GRAM POSITIVE AND GRAM
             ..NEGATIVE RODS,MODERATE GRAM NEGATIVE DIPLOCOCCI.
             ..ABUNDANT CELLS ? OF TYPE
       CULTURE:
       ABUNDANT STAPH AUREUS
          PEN R    METH S    ERYTH S    CEPH S    TETRA S
          CHLOR S
       VERY SCANT NORMAL THROAT FLORA PRESENT

04/08  SPUTUM    SN:5277
####   FINAL REPORT:
       SMEAR..READ BY DOCTOR
       CULTURE:
       ABUNDANT STAPH AUREUS
       SEE EARLIER CULTURE FOR SENSITIVITIES
       NORMAL THROAT FLORA ABSENT
```

```
04/09    SPUTUM     SN:5534
         VERY RARE PROTEUS SPECIES..OVERGROWING CULTURE
         ABUNDANT GRAM NEGATIVE RODS
            CEPH R     TETRA S     CHLOR I     AMP S     STREP S
            KANA S     GENTA S     COLI S
         ? OF ABUNDANT STAPH SPECIES
```

Figure 4-6d The next day at 4 p.m. no new data is available on SN:5534 but other cultures have been finalized.

```
04/12/72    12N MGH                    WHITE,THOMAS F    GR3AS    76-60-72



                    ----SPUTUM

04/08    SPUTUM    SN:5184
####     FINAL REPORT:
            SMEAR..ABUNDANT GRAM POSITIVE COCCI IN PAIRS.CHAINS AND
               ..CLUSTERS. ABUNDANT SMALL GRAM POSITIVE AND GRAM
               ..NEGATIVE RODS.MODERATE GRAM NEGATIVE DIPLOCOCCI.
               ..ABUNDANT CELLS ? OF TYPE
            CULTURE:
            ABUNDANT STAPH AUREUS
               PEN R     METH S     ERYTH S     CEPH S     TETRA S
            CHLOR S
            VERY SCANT NORMAL THROAT FLORA PRESENT

04/08    SPUTUM    SN:5277
####     FINAL REPORT:
            SMEAR: READ BY DOCTOR
            CULTURE:
            ABUNDANT STAPH AUREUS
            SEE EARLIER CULTURE FOR SENSITIVITIES
            NORMAL THROAT FLORA ABSENT

04/09    SPUTUM    SN:5534
####     FINAL REPORT:
            VERY RARE PROTEUS MIRABILIS..OVERGROWING CULTURE
            ABUNDANT HERELLEA
               CEPH R     TETRA S     CHLOR I     AMP S     STREP S
               KANA S     GENTA S     COLI S
            ABUNDANT STAPH AUREUS
            SEE EARLIER CULTURE FOR SENSITIVITIES
```

Figure 4-6e At noon on the second day the report is finalized on SN:5534 with the addition of species identification.

those who wish to adapt the programs to systems using MUMPS. An experienced MUMPS programmer spent about 400 hours studying changes that would be required to execute these MGH programs through a PDP-15 computer dedicated to other MUMPS operations in use by our laboratory. He concluded that it would be easier to write new programs than to make the required changes.

The MGH System takes advantage of an interface with a clinical chemistry reporting system and a medical records system that assists in the rapid recognition of patients from the previous entry of history numbers, patient names, and locations. This provides one of the first advantages of a computer information system. It controls the association of incorrect names and history numbers, minimizes confusion of patients with similar names, and keeps track of patients as they are transferred and discharged. All information is entered through an alpha-numeric keyboard. The developers believe that this mode of entry results in fewer errors than matrix type keyboards, punched cards, or marked sense cards. [Recently light sensitive probes used with cathode ray tube (CRT) displays have been introduced in some laboratories for entering data. These may carry the same risk of erroneous entry as do cards. Regardless of the method of entry most systems utilize some feedback which requires verification.] After assessioning a series of bacteriology specimens, the MGH System prints individualized workcards which provide an outline for entering observations on smears and media that are ordinarily examined for each type of specimen. As work is conducted by technologists, they present the results to terminal operators who enter it through an alpha-numeric keyboard on a CRT terminal. All frequently used terms, such as bacterial species names and common phrases, are abbreviated or otherwise coded. Entry of the proper abbreviated symbols results in the eventual appearance of the completed name or phrase which is then verified by the person entering the data. This system contains an almost unlimited capacity for free language entry, an important feature in bacteriology reporting.

This is a real time system which allows telephone inquiries to the laboratory to be handled by a clerk who enters the name of the patient and immediately receives a display of all information that has been entered. Technologists are usually not disturbed for information that may be on their workcards because the economy of effort expended on entering preliminary results usually insures that there is no new data that has not been incorporated into the system. Certain unique features of this system provide the technologist with an easy method for entering such information. At midnight on the day of receipt of blood and urine cultures, the system automatically changes a report of "pending" to "negative to date" and "no significant growth," respectively. Technologists examine these specimens in the morning and enter evidence of growth observed on blood cultures and urine cultures. The system produces lists, by patient care units, of the status of all blood and urine cultures twice a day. This procedure was dropped when patient reports were increased from once to twice daily. This has eliminated most of the telephone calls, because the majority of requests related to bloods and urines. It insures rapid entry of results by technologists because they recognize that until an entry is made the system carries a report of "pending" or "negative to date." The computer provides a list for the chief bacteriologist of all specimens on which no report is rendered within 48 hours. Technologists gain pride from keeping their specimens off the list, which has become progressively shorter.

Twice each day updated reports are prepared by a line printer in the laboratory. These are sent to the various patient care units. Once a week all of this data is reorganized in the computer file and a weekly summary is printed, organizing reports on all specimens received during that week by type and in chronological order. This offers little advantage to the patient who is hospitalized for a few days and has one or two cultures taken. It does provide an enormous advantage in the evaluation of charts for the many patients who have been admitted for extended periods.

The MGH program employs a number of special applications in antimicrobial susceptibility testing. These include automatic scanning of antimicrobial zone diameters, which are interpreted by the computer using Bauer-Kirby break points. Results are stored and printed on the patient's report with other information entered by technologists. Storage of this data has made it possible to prepare computer printed distributions of zone diameters for various species. Although this data can be used for quality control, it is primarily of academic interest. The system also produces clinically useful periodic profiles of susceptibility to various antimicrobials. Special programs have been developed to compare the precision and accuracy of the visual reading of zone diameters by students and technologists with the results obtained by the automatic scanner. This provides a form of internal quality control and maintenance of skills which would prove essential if the scanner went "down" and the customary visual inspection of zones of inhibition were required.

Other automatic data systems are being developed for specific microbiologic functions. Petralli and his associates have developed systems for comparing zone diameter values obtained with individual isolates to a file of data collected on previous isolates of the same species (1). Applying Bayes theorem to this data allowed these workers to detect errors in 12–15% of the reports. These consisted of errors in identification, measurement of zone diameters, mixed cultures, and technical errors in the performance of the disk test. A lower percentage of errors (6–8%) has been detected in the author's laboratory using a system that analyzes profiles of susceptibility, but does not incorporate actual zone diameter measurements.

An obvious potential application for computers in bacteriology is speciation by automatic analysis of morphologic, serologic, and biochemical data.

Its possible value has led to some controversy. Some authorities believe that the number of occasions when a computer would be required to provide speciation are too few to make the system economical. Furthermore, the analysis of results obtained with unusual isolates provides an intellectual challenge, which affords an important escape from some of the more routine aspects of day to day work. A large centralized file of morphologic and biochemical data representing the cumulative experience of major centers, such as the CDC, could be of considerable value in identifying unusual isolates. The author's laboratory is evaluating the use of such a program, which was developed elsewhere but is accessible on a time sharing basis, for less than a dollar per use, to anyone with a teletype and a phone coupler. Identical standards of interpretation, media, and biochemical tests are essential if the results are to be valid. Gavan has shown that speciation based on the usual random process of inspecting reference tables would be qualified substantially by differences in statistical probability that are ordinarily not recognized (2). Some investigators have suggested that bacteria not be identified by computer, but that the computer be used to verify the use of minimum criteria and the validity of reports. This involves the entry of a much larger amount of data than a simple assessioning and reporting system would handle.

A number of quality control functions might prove useful. Reports on sources of specimens that are improperly submitted could be prepared. If this could have been established for all of the inferior quality specimens submitted to us and listed in Figure 4-3, it would have been possible for us to investigate improper practices before the problem reached such proportions that physicians complained about it. Automatic accounting of workloads is easily accomplished. A system used in the author's laboratory is in Chapter 5.

Control of precision and accuracy of the disk susceptibility test of Bauer et al. is assisted by several computer applications in the author's laboratory. These are described in Chapter 6.

Computers can be effectively applied to the processing of infection control data. A number of institutions, including that of the author, code data on patients with hospital associated infections. Periodic reports indicating the attack rate for various types of infections are generated by services and locations within the hospital. The etiologic agents are listed in decreasing order of frequency. The author and other workers interested in hospital associated infections have speculated on the potential value of identifying cross infections by computer identification of unique susceptibility patterns on patient care units. No experience has been published regarding the application of such a system. Two outbreaks of cross infection were detected by technologists in the Hartford Hospital through the observation of unique susceptibility patterns. One case concerned a *Serratia sp.* and the other a *Klebsiella pneumoniae* isolated from a number of patients on the same unit.

DATE 09/30/72   PERIOD ENDING 09/30/72

	TOTAL PATIENTS DISCHARGED	PATIENTS WITH INFECTIONS	TOTAL NUMBER OF INFECTIONS	PATNT WITH INFEC PRES ON ADM.	INFECTIONS PRESENT ON ADM.	PATNT WITH HOSP ASSOC INFECTIONS	HOSPITAL ASSOCIATED INFECTIONS
MEDICINE	8427	251 (3)	317 (4)	251 (3)	317 (4)	251 (3)	317 (4)
SURGERY	7079	378 (5)	491 (7)	378 (5)	491 (7)	378 (5)	491 (7)
OBSTETRICS	3564	38 (1)	41 (1)	38 (1)	41 (1)	38 (1)	41 (1)
PEDIATRICS	3311	15 ( )	15 ( )	15 ( )	15 ( )	15 ( )	15 ( )
EYE-EAR-NOSE-THROAT	1192	3 ( )	3 ( )	3 ( )	3 ( )	3 ( )	3 ( )
NEUROSURGERY	1278	116 (9)	164 (13)	116 (9)	164 (13)	116 (9)	164 (13)
ORTHOPEDICS	2168	72 (3)	90 (4)	72 (3)	90 (4)	72 (3)	90 (4)
UROLOGY	2050	78 (4)	93 (5)	78 (4)	93 (5)	78 (4)	93 (5)
GYNECOLOGY	4106	155 (4)	166 (4)	155 (4)	166 (4)	155 (4)	166 (4)
ALL SERVICES	33175	1106 (3)	1380 (4)	1106 (3)	1380 (4)	1106 (3)	1380 (4)

HOSPITAL ASSOCIATED INFECTIONS

MEDICINE

RESPIRATORY INFECTIONS

    28 TOPOGRAPHY   75

        ETIOLOGY   CASES

UNKNOWN	29
KLEBSIELLA	21
PSEUD AERUG	11
S. AUREUS	8
E. COLI	6
ENTEROBACTER	5
PROTEUS	5
D. PNEUMONIAE	5
SERRATIA	3
H. FLU	3
STREP PYOGENES	1

        TOTALS   97

SEPTICEMIAS

    OX TOPOGRAPHY   41

        ETIOLOGY   CASES

E. COLI	12
ENTEROBACTER	7
PSEUD AERUG	6
KLEBSIELLA	5
S. AUREUS	4
SERRATIA	3
S. EPIDERM	2
STREP FAECALIS	2
PROTEUS	1
BACTERCIDES	1
D. PNEUMONIAE	1
STREP PYOGENES	1
MICRO ANAER	1

        TOTALS   46

```
URINARY TRACT INFECTIONS

   70 TOPOGRAPHY        1553  MORPHOLOGY                    199

        ETIOLOGY                                         CASES


     E. COLI                                              98
     PROTEUS                                              28
     KLEBSIELLA                                           25
     PSEUD AERUG                                          24
     ENTEROBACTER                                         15
     STREP FAECALIS                                       13
     CANDIDA                                              11
     SERRATIA                                              7
     CITROBACTER                                           2
     S. EPIDERM                                            2
     XANTHOMONAS                                           1
     HERELLEA                                              1


        TOTALS                                          227
```

Figure 4-7 A portion of the surveillance report of hospital associated infections. Note the arrangement by computer of etiologic agents in descending order of frequency. Such data is helpful for guiding physicians in the prevention and treatment of such infections.

One commercial organization is in business to process and report antimicrobial susceptibility data and infection control information for hospitals. Further discussion of the first area is found in Chapter 6 (p. 153). Infection control data was distorted by the tabulation of *isolates* instead of *infections*, a practice that could lead to the impression that an outbreak had occurred when in fact multiple isolates had been received from the same patient. This has been corrected, but representatives of the company concede that the results are no better than the data entered. This is affected by large differences in efficiency and standards for defining hospital associated infections in various hospitals. Workers in institutions that possess their own computer services have established that purchasing these programs is more costly than conducting it themselves. It is doubtful that incorporating individual hospital data into national statistics derived from institutions using widely varying standards is worth the added cost. The CDC has been conducting a survey of nosocomial infections in a number of hospitals. These data are being processed by computer and the program is limited to institutions with which the CDC could establish close coordination of standards.

CHAPTER 5

Workloads, Space, and Personnel

SOCIOECONOMIC FACTORS

The largest obstacle to developing quality control programs in most clinical laboratories is an excessive workload and an inadequate number of sufficiently trained personnel. The experience of those engaged in allied health training suggests that existing programs are coming closer than ever to meeting current demands for technicians and technologists. This conflicts with observations reported by the University of Connecticut in 1967, forecasting a need in Connecticut for more than 1000 additional medical laboratory technicians by 1976 (1). One reason for these differences is fluctuating economic conditions. In 1965 the average duration of employment for personnel in the author's laboratory was 1.8 years. By 1972 this had increased 55% to 2.8 years. The economic conditions of the last several years have caused more female laboratory personnel to continue working although a somewhat larger number are now married and gain financial support from their husbands. There has also been a greater tendency to return to full or part-time employment following childbirth. These factors have reduced the demand for graduates. On the other hand, we are aware of numerous laboratories throughout the country in which 10% of their personnel or less have had formal training in laboratory science. These institutions are not expressing a demand for graduates of accredited programs for two reasons: their turnover rate has decreased, and their salary structures are not sufficiently competitive to attract trained laboratory personnel.

	Highly Proficient		Capable		Inadequately Skilled		Total
Pathologist	13	15%	63	72%	12	14%	88
Microbiologist	39	60%	25	39%	1	2%	65
Supervisor	35	43%	42	52%	4	5%	81
Technologists	25	27%	59	63%	10	11%	94
Night workers	4	5%	53	63%	27	32%	84

Figure 5-1 Appraisal by pathologists of the adequacy of the skills of their staff in clinical microbiology in 86 laboratories. The dependency of pathologists on microbiologists and supervisors is reflected in this data.

It is uncertain how rapidly licensure and other regulations governing the activities of laboratory workers will be introduced. Although these regulations may force the employment of better qualified individuals in some laboratories, they inevitably result in arbitrary restrictions that interfere with the organization and efficient use of personnel in properly staffed laboratories. Increasing public pressure due to rising hospital costs will not improve the prospects of competitive salary scales for trained laboratory workers in many institutions. The threat or fact of unionization will improve the economic status of laboratory workers, but may also introduce undesired constraints on the efficient utilization of personnel.

It is not possible to develop all of these problems and to propose solutions here. These remarks serve only to draw attention to the effects of limited personnel qualifications on high quality performance (Figure 5-1). All technical personnel should participate in continuing education programs. These should be conducted once a month within individual institutions (Figure 5-2). All workers should have an opportunity to attend an annual program within the state. Senior personnel should attend an annual meeting of a major laboratory organization. Expenses should be reimbursed and time from work excused.

	Regional or National Program (once per year) (%)	Intramural Program (once per month) (%)
Pathologist	92	56
Microbiologist	84	56
Supervisor	76	49
Technologist	46	34

Figure 5-2 Continuing education activity of various personnel in 86 microbiology laboratories. Technologists should attend monthly intramural and yearly regional programs. Supervisors and microbiologists should attend at least one national meeting annually.

WORKLOADS

There is widespread recognition that standards for measuring workloads vary greatly among laboratories. Bacteriology workloads are often expressed by the total number of *tests* performed rather than *specimens* received. Although enumerating *tests* may reflect an increase in the complexity of work with more accuracy than enumerating *specimens*, the lack of standardization precludes comparison with other laboratories. A review of workloads, computed by participants in workshops conducted by the author, revealed 52 laboratories in which less than 4500 specimens were processed per equivalent full-time worker per year (Figure 5-3). Thirty-four laboratories exceeded this workload. A workload of 4500 specimens per year per worker has been maintained in bacteriology at Hartford Hospital since 1965. In making this computation it is necessary to include those workers who directly process specimens. This excludes clerks, secretaries, media preparation technicians, and the portion of the supervisor's time that is primarily administrative. The performance of nonbacteriologic tests by personnel affects target workload values. Including serologic procedures, urinalysis, and other body fluid analyses increases productivity. In the author's laboratory where these other procedures are performed in the Microbiology Division, the overall workload is maintained at 6500 specimens per worker per year.

In a more recent study we reviewed the staffing and workloads of 27 institutions with proficient microbiology laboratories directed by recognized clinical microbiologists and pathologists. Twenty-one of these laboratories were situated in university hospitals whereas most of the 86 laboratories included in the older survey were community hospitals. Only one of these laboratories was not directed by a Ph.D. or M.D. specialist in clinical microbiology. The number of budgeted hours per week was divided by 40 to obtain the equivalent number of nondoctoral microbiologists, supervisors,

	Mean (%)	Range (%)	Hartford Hospital (%)
Diagnostic	70	50–90	52
Education	10	5–20	12
Development and Q.C.	5	0–15	6
Collection	5	0–15	5
Nonproduction	5	0–10	15
Administration	5	2–15	10

Figure 5-3 Distribution of working hours among various functions in 66 microbiology laboratories. Note the substantial amount of time spent on functions other than diagnostic work, which is not reflected in the usual accounting of workloads by specimens received or processed.

Specimens per Worker per Year	Labs
Less than 1500	2
1500–2000	6
2000–2500	2 } 15
2500–3000	7
3000–3500	1
3500–4000	2
4000–4500	2
4500–5000	2
More than 5000	2

Figure 5-4 Number of specimens processed per worker per year in 27 proficient microbiology laboratories. Workers included nondoctoral microbiologists, supervisors, technicians (including evening and night personnel), clerks, and secretaries. Workers exclude doctoral staff, media preparation, research, development, and education personnel.

technicians (including evening and night), clerks, and secretaries. Doctoral staff, media preparation, research and development, and education staff were excluded. Most of the laboratories demonstrated workloads between 1500 and 3000 specimens per worker per year (Figure 5-4). Utilizing this definition the author's laboratory is operating at 2700 specimens per worker per year in bacteriology.

Rappaport observed a median of 10,000 tests per technologist for all laboratory work in a survey of 88 hospitals published in 1960 (2). Unfortunately this figure has been applied by hospital administrators to laboratory workers in general, without the recognition that workloads of less than one half of this amount should not be exceeded in bacteriology.

Laboratory directors have been frustrated by the inability to measure workloads incurred by activities other than diagnostic services as a basis for substantiating requests for increases in personnel. Useful data was obtained from 66 of 86 community hospital laboratories indicating that only about 70% of the time was spent on diagnostic work. The remainder was applied to education, development, quality control, administration, and collection of specimens. Laboratory directors estimated that about 5% of employee time was nonproductive. Obviously it is not possible to add the hours spent on this type of work to the number of specimens received and obtain any kind of useful number. Effort expended on diagnostic work must be translated into hours. This may be accomplished by studying a period during which adequate laboratory staffing is observed. If staffing is consistently inadequate, calculations must be based on hypothetical conditions. Specimens received may be multiplied by the unit values established for charging purposes. The total number of units performed is divided into the number of actual hours or minutes worked minus the time spent on nondiagnostic and nonproductive activity. This provides a baseline time/work constant for *minutes* of work required to produce one *unit* of work. Thus the laboratory director may plot a computed workload based on hours spent on nondiagnostic activities added to diagnostic work and calculated by multiplying the time/work constant by the number of units of diagnostic work performed. If the total of actual hours worked is plotted simultaneously, it is possible to illustrate graphically any increase in computed work relative to actual hours worked. Such a system has been used in our laboratory since 1966. A more detailed description of the computations is reported elsewhere (3).

In 1972 this system was improved through use of the College of American Pathologists Workload Reporting System (4). We were gratified to observe that the time/work units developed for this system agreed very closely with those developed in our own laboratory. Thus the standards incorporated in this system agree closely with our impression of appropriate workload conditions in bacteriology. It is not necessary to incorporate a separate estimate of nonproductive time when using the CAP system because this has been incorporated into the time/work units.

It is an established management principle that a maximum of 85% of budgeted hours will be in use at any time. This results from sick-time, vacations, and unfilled positions. It is necessary to take this into consideration when discussing needs for budgeted hours based on computation of workloads.

In the author's laboratory a variety of workload reporting sheets have been developed for use in various sections including the media preparation room (Figure 5-5). Each day personnel enter totals for each item listed. Time spent on nondiagnostic work is recorded on special accounting forms that are filled out and submitted by each worker once a week. A program was developed for entering this data, including time card totals, via teletype into a real time automatic data system. The program incorporates sufficient controls to prevent unintentional omission or reentry of data. The computer file contains all of the unit values required to compute the CAP Workload Reporting System. At the end of each accounting period, which occurs every 28 days, the system produces a one page report that summarizes budgeted hours, actual hours of work performed, and the computed workload. This is plotted graphically to provide a continuous estimate of increasing work and the need for increases in budgeted hours (Figure 5-6).

Other laboratory divisions in the Hartford Hospital are not using such a workload reporting system and continue to depend on changes in total specimens received. For this reason the system has been programmed to produce similar lists of specimens received by microbiology for incorporation into general laboratory accounting reports. The previous manual method of conducting this entire activity for the microbiology division required about 40 hours of clerk time per accounting period. The new system has reduced this to 10 hours per accounting period. In addition a marked increase in efficiency has been observed. About 10% of our workload was

SHEET A

Bacteriology Sheet

Date:___*SepTembeR 30, 1972*_____

Daily Total	Sun.	Mon.	Tues.	Wed.	Thurs.	Fri.	Sat.
1. Blood cultures	38	40	36	46	83	55	60
2. Urine cultures	65	37	56	104	64	50	49
3. Throat cultures	12	5	8	14	15	22	24
4. Sputum cultures	21	10	13	19	23	18	15
5. Wound cultures	16	11	9	23	23	20	16
6. Fluid cultures	20	10	6	17	21	19	22
7. Feces cultures	5	6	6	10	8	3	4
8. Hospital control	0	0	0	0	18	2	0
9. Tube dilution	0	0	0	0	0	0	0
10. Serum inhibitory	0	0	0	0	0	0	0
11. Misc. Gram stains	4	2	0	2	5	2	0
12. Darkfield exam	0	0	0	0	1	0	0
13. Gram stains	19	22	37	42	42	50	53
Slide coagulase	7	9	5	13	10	10	11
Serologic Agglut.	0	3	0	0	16	19	0

ADDENDUM: For Blood Cultures, count aerobic and anaerobic cultures individually.

Figure 5-5 (*a*) Example of workload recording sheet for bacteriology. The CAP workload reporting system is used.

not being recorded by the previous manual system because of its cumbersome nature, demands on clerical time, and lack of control over omissions in recording work performed.

In some laboratories the problem is not managing and documenting excessive workloads but maintaining sufficient work in microbiology to assure quality performance. As the volume of microbiology decreases, the percentage of quality control activity becomes larger. This is discussed in greater depth in Chapter 6. It is possible to reach a point at which each use of a particular medium, biochemical test, or serologic procedure requires concurrent quality control with cultures, antigens, or antisera of known reactivity. It is impossible to define at what point laboratories should desist from doing microbiology. It is questionable whether performance can be maintained at proficient levels if less than one specimen per week is received for culture of blood, spinal fluid, feces, throat, sputum, or urine.

The quality of clinical microbiology provided in areas of heavy population concentration, such as exists on the American eastern seaboard, could be improved greatly if laboratories performing such small volumes of microbiology referred specimens to larger conveniently accessible laboratories. Institutional pride frequently stands in the way of such arrangements. A different problem is encountered in western portions of the United States where the only alternative to performing small volumes of microbiology is mailing specimens, with the associated risk of deterioration and delay in reporting. We hope that the current obsession with laboratory proficiency

		Sun.	Mon.	Tues.	Wed.	Thurs.	Fri.	Sat.
	NAME _Sally Jones_ Week of (Date of Sunday) _Oct. 1, 1972_							
	I. EDUCATION	/////	/////	/////	/////	/////	/////	/////
	A. TEACHING	/////	/////	/////	/////	/////	/////	/////
1.	a. Workshop							
2.	b. Bench			↑	6°	6^c	6^c	
3.	c. Preparation							
	B. TRAINING	/////	/////	/////	/////	/////	/////	/////
4.	a. Workshop							
5.	b. Bench							
	C. LECTURES	/////	/////	/////	/////	/////	/////	/////
6.	a. Med. Tech.			L				
7.	b. Conferences			OFF				
8.	c. Other (specify)							
	II. ADMINISTRATION	/////	/////	/////	/////	/////	/////	/////
9.	A. SUPERVISION							
	B. MEETINGS	/////	/////	/////	/////	/////	/////	/////
10.	a. Department			DAY				
11.	b. Misc.(Specify)			OFF				
12.	C. SCHEDULE							
13.	D. ORDERING							
14.	E. OTHER (specify)							
15.	III. PROJECTS (specify)							
	IV. SPECIAL SERVICES	/////	/////	/////	/////	/////	/////	/////
16.	A. QUALITY CONTROL		$1/4$		$1/4^o$ media	$1/4^o$ media	$3/4^o$ media	
17.	B. OTHER							
18.	V. COLLECTION Round off to 1/4 hr.		$1 1/4^o$		$3/4^o$	$1/2^o$	1^c	

Figure 5-5 (*b*) Extra time report submitted weekly by each worker to indicate time spent on tasks other than diagnostic work.

```
        BACTERIOLOGY              PERIOD #1        FROM 10/1/72 THRU 10/28/72


                              PER. TOTAL            ACCUM.

    BLOOD CULTURES              689                  689

    URINE CULTURES            1,409                1,409

    THROAT CULTURES            447                  447

    SPUTUM CULTURE             431                  431

    WOUND CULTURES             499                  499

    FLUID CULTURES             497                  497

    FECES CULTURES             182                  182

    HOSPITAL CONT'L            119                  119

    TUBE DILUTION                1                    1

    SERUM INHIB                 14                   14

    MISC. GRAM STAINS           96                   96

    DARKFIELD EXAM               1                    1

    AFB SMEARS ONLY             27                   27

    AFB CULTURES               103                  103

    MYCOLOGY CULTURES           60                   60

    MYCOLOGY SMEARS             71                   71
                                                   .....


            TOTAL            4,655                4,655
                                                  ......
```

Figure 5-5 (c)   Computer printed list of specimens received.

does not result in the discontinuation of services in areas where this may have a more adverse effect on patient care than the availability of some kind of a laboratory, albeit substandard.

SPACE

The laboratory director who solves his personnel shortage may find himself with an overcrowded laboratory. What is the minimum amount of space that should be allotted to each worker? There are several ways to measure

```
        MICROBIOLOGY ACCOUNTING DATA IN HOURS FOR PERIOD #1

                  10/1/72 THRU 10/28/72

        TITLE                HOURS       HOURS      CUM/CATEG       HOURS

 I.  BUDGETED HOURS.............................................................4,900

 II. HOURS NEEDED (CALC.)......................................................5,283

      A. NON-PRODUCTION..................

      B. COLLECTION.....................      264         264

      C. NON-DIAGNOSTIC.................    1,234       1,498

           1. EDUCATION.......    515

           2. ADMINISTRATION..    270

           3. PROJECTS........      2

           4. SPECIAL SERVICES.  448

      D. DIAGNOSTIC WORKLOAD.............    3,785       5,283

           1. TECHNICAL......   3,097

           2. CLERICAL.......     688

 III. HOURS WORKED.............................................................4,665

      A. REGULAR.....................    4,466       4,466

      B. OVERTIME....................      199       4,665

      C. SICK-TIME...................      130       4,795

      D. HOLIDAY.....................       40       4,835

      E. EXCUSED.....................       26       4,860

      F. ABSENT......................        2       4,862

      G. VACATION....................      184       5,046

      H. IN TRAINING.................        0       5,046
```

Figure 5-5 (*d*) Summary data printed by computer to allow easy comparison of budgeted hours, actual hours worked, and hours needed based on the CAP workload reporting system criteria. Regular hours worked was 4446. The 199 hours of overtime worked reflects a lack of adequate staffing to handle a workload calculated at 5283. Budgeted hours of 4900 must be increased. This type of objective analysis becomes increasingly necessary when negotiating budgets with hospital administrations who must be able to justify any charges to third party payers and government commissions.

November 15, 1973

MEMORANDUM

To: R. S. Beckett, M.D.

From: R. C. Bartlett, M.D.

Subject: Personnel hours in Microbiology

_____

We continue to experience a gradual increase in specimens which are received for processing in Microbiology. In addition we have made a number of improvements which we regard to be significant contributions to improved patient care. These changes have been introduced cautiously with careful review of practices and policies prevailing in other institutions. Unfortunately these improvements have required expenditure of more time on many specimens. Examples are:

1. 1969- Repeat of 15% of total isolates speciated and tested for sensitivities because of quality control detection of deviations from expected results suggesting error. 4-6% of total are proven to be erroneous and report is corrected.

2. 1969- Preparation of trichome stains for intestinal protozoa. More time consuming system for concentration of ova.

3. 1969- Antinuclear factor procedure according to method of Rothfield.

4. 1970- Routine anaerobic culture culture in addition to aerobic culture on all bloods submitted (doubled workload for blood cultures).

5. 1971-72- Addition of new media and biochemical tests for more reliable identification of Streptococcus pyogenes, Neisseria gonorrhoeae, Bacteroides sp. and Streptococcus sp.

6. 1971- Cummulative report system in December 1971.

7. 1972- A system for detection of poor quality specimens from the lower respiratory tract; limited bacteriology is performed and repeat specimens are requested.

8. 1972- Routine quality control testing of all media and biochemicals before use.

9. 1972- Complete revision of mycology methods with transfer of 20 hours to diagnostic services from development

10. 1972- Isolation, speciation and sensitivity testing of all Bacteroides isolates.

11. 1972- Daily delivery of results of throat cultures
on children received during previous 24 hours to
Pediatric clinic by 10 am.

Simultaneously we have introduced measures to reduce irrelevant
or redundant work and work on specimens of poor quality. This has
required development of policies which have progressively reduced
arbitrary and inefficient use of our services. This has been associated with complaints from some physicians that our service has de-
teriorated. Examples of policies introduced to control work are:

1. 1969- Request consultations when requests are non-
specific or inappropriate for the type of specimen.

2. 1969- Reporting of Strep pyogenes only from throats

3. 1969- Refer all CSF serologies to State Lab.

4. 1969- Request repeat urine specimens for culture when
three or more species are isolated.

5. 1970- Refusal of duplicate specimens submitted same
day.

6. 1970- Refusal of specimens submitted during night for
which technician is not called.

7. 1970- Do not repeat antibiotic susceptibility test on
isolates from same site within 4 days.

8. 1971- Request repeat specimens of urine when time of
collection is not shown or delay of more than 4 hours
occurs in transit.

9. 1971- Discontinue Rhodamine-auramine stains on tissues.

10. 1972- Performance of certain tests on selected days
only instead of Monday-Friday.

Discussion

1. Continued increases in numbers of specimens submitted and ac-
commodation of selected requests for new services will require tighter
controls on utilization if existing standards of quality are to be
maintained without increases in personnel. Our policies for controlled
utilization have been presented at several national meetings where
substantial numbers of participants:

    a. were not sure the constraints were justifiable
    b. had applied few if any of them in their own institutions
    c. did not think their medical staffs would accept them

2. Several observations contribute to an evaluation of increased
work in their division.

    a. A 10% increase in specimens received has occurred
since the last increase in budgeted hours in 1969

    b. Overtime persists at about 40 hours per week

c. A workload computation system developed by us and
used until last year showed a 6% increase in work
between 1968 and 1972.

d. A workload reporting system developed by the College
of American Pathologists and programmed by us for
our MUMPS-IOL data system has shown a 13% increase in
work during the past year. Part of this is a result
of increased efficiency and organization resulting
from the automatic data system approach. We know of
several areas in which workload recording was not
conducted during the last two years because of confusion and dissatisfaction with previous accounting
methods. Note that the workload appeared to decline
by total specimens received (A) and computation (D)
during this interval. C is budgeted hours. Subscript
1 and 2 denotes before and after including clerical
and secretarial work and hours.

e. A projected slope for computed work (E) shows an increase
of 40% in contrast to the 10% increase in specimens (B).
This suggests a more dramatic increase in effort expended
per specimen than we have implied in the list of improvements in service provided above.

Conclusion

A 10% increase in budgeted hours appears justifiable from observation
of growth in work in this division. This represents 100 hours/week. A request for 40 clerk hours has been made and may be included in this amount.
60 hours for technicians grades I-III was placed in the 1972-73 planning
budget. We wish to request authorization for use of these hours.

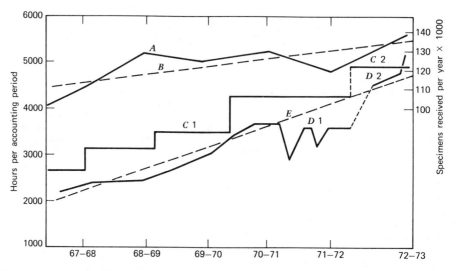

Figure 5-6 Memorandum containing supporting data for request for additional man-hours.
This demonstrates the extensive documentation that hospital administrators require because
of intense competition for funds among hospital departments.

laboratory space. Architects and hospital administrators usually think in terms of *gross* square feet. This is obtained by measuring the outside dimensions of a building or one of its component wings. This includes walls, corridors, elevators, and utilities. *Net* square feet is usable space. This excludes walls, corridors, elevators, utilities, and staircases. It is obtained by measuring the inside dimensions of an office or laboratory room. It should include space occupied by benches and equipment. *Gross* square footage is almost always one and one half times *net* square footage. Conversely *net* square footage may be obtained by taking two thirds of the *gross* square footage. To compound matters, third parties, such as Blue Cross, may request square footage figures taken to the midpoint of exterior walls.

In the author's survey of 86 community hospital laboratories, an average of 120 net ft^2 per person with a range from 40 to 350 net ft^2 was reported in bacteriology. Our laboratory has decreased from 75 to 60 net ft^2 per worker during the past 5 years. Although personnel gradually accommodate to increasingly crowded conditions, activities are significantly encumbered below 75 net ft^2 per worker (Figure 5-7). Problems include disorganization in assembling and processing materials, failure to refer to requisition and report cards because of insufficient space for arranging these documents, contamination hazards resulting from dropping or breaking plates and tubes that had been stacked or placed in precarious positions, and interpersonal conflict resulting from noise and mutual interference in the organization and conduct of work.

In 1960 Rappaport referred to work published by Grey who recommended 110 net ft^2 for persons engaged in administrative activities. One hundred fifty ft^2 was recommended for executive personnel and 230 net ft^2 per person was considered a minimum in laboratories. The National Research Council of Canada concluded that 280 usable or net ft^2 per person should be established as a standard for planning purposes (2). In Rappaport's survey of 80 hospitals a range of 120–170 net ft^2 per technologist was observed with a median value of 152 net ft^2. When all employees were considered, a range of 98–128 net ft^2 per employee was found with a mean of 114 net ft^2.

Grey's recommendations include space for future expansion and do not represent a minimum standard for occupancy. On the basis of these observations we have selected 100 net ft^2 per worker as a minimum (Figure 5-8).

Laboratory directors must establish objective methods for computing the adequacy of existing space and future space needs. Use of the standards presented in this chapter should make it possible to determine whether a microbiology laboratory is adequately staffed for the workload and whether sufficient space is available (Figure 5-9). If there is insufficient staff one may compute the extent of crowding that would occur if a sufficient staff were available. When computing occupancy it is important not to utilize the

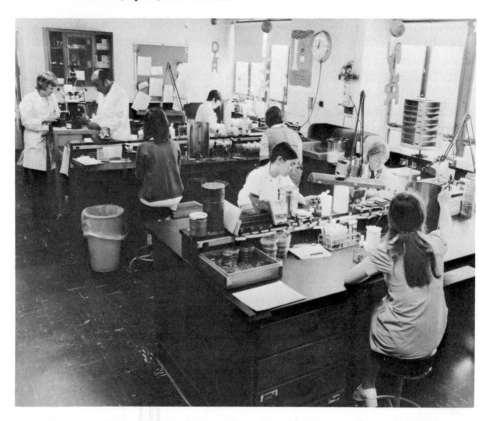

Figure 5-7 A portion of Hartford Hospital Microbiology Laboratory showing six technologists using 460 ft^2 (75 net ft^2 per worker). This exceeds the recommended utilization of 100 net ft^2 per worker. Cheryl Rutz, technical supervisor, and George Carrington, microbiologist, are shown making laboratory rounds using a portable microscope table. (Photograph by the author.)

total number of full-time equivalent employees but a number representing the maximum simultaneous occupancy. Employees who are assigned to weekends and holidays take days off to compensate for this. Other employees are assigned to evening and night shifts. Vacations and sick time reduce somewhat the number of people who are simultaneously present. Over an extended period we have observed that simultaneous occupancy averages 75% of the number of full-time employees.

Hospital administrators must allocate expanded space to departments that provide the most compelling data to support their future needs. In the absence of such data there is a tendency to underestimate the increasing growth of laboratory work and to hope that increased productivity will accommodate it. A baseline of at least 10 years growth is required to allow projection of space needs for 10 years hence. This is a minimum target for planning because it takes about that long to establish funding, prepare drawings, and complete major hospital construction. Growth should be plotted on both arithmetic and semilogarithmic graph paper. If growth is

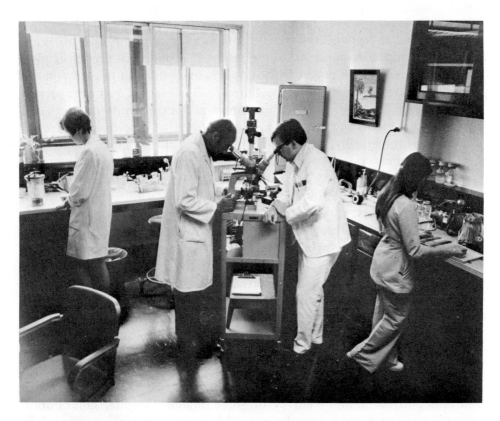

Figure 5-8 Part of the Hartford Hospital Microbiology Laboratory showing two technologists using 210 net ft^2 illustrating the maximum utilization of space for efficient operation. George Carrington, microbiologist, and Victor Wylie, pathology resident, are shown making laboratory rounds with a portable table equipped with a double headed microscope useful for teaching and reviewing the interpretation of observations on problem specimens. (Photograph by the author.)

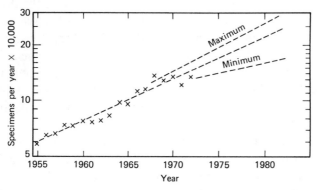

Figure 5-9 Projection of the workload in microbiology based on specimens received. Growth appears to be a semilogarithmic function. A curve that is difficult to extrapolate is obtained on arithmetic graph paper. Dotted lines were established in 1965 on the basis of the previous 10 years' experience. Note the close approximation of actual increase in work with extrapolation through 1972. Such projections are essential for future planning of personnel and space needs.

increasing at an exponential rate it produces a straight line on semi-logarithmic paper. A parabolic curve results if exponential growth is plotted on arithmetic graph paper. Obviously it is more difficult to extrapolate a curve than a straight line. Differences are usually observed only over periods of 5 –10 years. Plots of growth over shorter periods often do not display a clearly arithmetic or logarithmic increase. (Note that growth in Figure 5-6 is plotted arithmetically. This period is included in the much longer projection plotted exponentially in Figure 5-9.) Alternatively, a mathematically computed projection could be made. This precise approach assumes that factors influencing the growth of laboratory work will remain constant. Socioeconomic pressures, automation, and screening are major factors that affect the rate of growth of laboratory work. It is certain that their impact will change dramatically over the next 10 years. This may appear to render futile any effort to project growth. The alternative is to accept increases in space of 25–50% based on an empirical allocation by hospital administration. Hospital administrators, third party payers, and the newly established hospital cost commissions express doubt that the exponential rate of growth will continue. The problem of controlled use of laboratory services has been discussed extensively elsewhere in this book. We believe that it is premature to assume that anyone but physicians who consume laboratory services can bring about a change in the rate of increase in utilization. In the author's survey of 86 community hospital laboratories, projection of space needs revealed a need for increases ranging from 10 to 100% in 5 years and from 30 to 400% in 10 years. Average estimates were 25% for 5 years and 100% for 10 years. In our laboratory we have estimated a need for a 40% increase in space in 5 years and a 100% increase in 10 years.

Data collected in our laboratory and displayed in Figure 5-6 indicate that a workload accounting system using relative values shows a more rapid increase in work performed than a system measuring only the number of specimens received. In our laboratory future workloads have been based on a projection of specimens only because other laboratory divisions do not use relative value systems for estimating workloads; and we have a 25 year base for projecting work based on specimens received. We are not sure whether a long range plot of relative value workload accounting data would produce the convenient and predictable straight line observed for specimen growth plotted on semilogarithmic paper.

Developing a second shift in the clinical laboratory has been proposed as a means of improving the efficiency of utilization and reducing future space needs. In many hospitals some personnel are assigned to other shifts to cover night, weekend, and holiday services. It is difficult to obtain qualified personnel to work at these hours and their supervision often presents a problem. Most institutions provide some pay differential for evenings, nights, and holidays. If this solution is proposed when negotiating space needs, administrators should be requested to compare the long term cost of providing a pay differential for evening shifts with the amortized cost of constructing new space. This demonstrates that construction of new space is more economical. Increasing emphasis on leisure time and anticipation of demands for larger pay differentials for work performed during these hours further detracts from any justification for this approach.

The following summary outlines an approach to projecting personnel and space needs:

1. Plot work over at least a 10 year period. Use specimens collected or data on workloads computed with relative values if available.
2. Determine whether the rate of growth is arithmetic or exponential. Plot on proper graph paper and extrapolate to 10 years hence.
3. Divide projected values of specimens collected by 4500 for bacteriology and by 6500 for inclusion of immunology, body fluids, and urinalysis. This provides the number of full-time personnel to perform diagnostic work. Add to this supervisors, clerks, secretaries, teaching, development, and quality control personnel, media production workers, and students including residents.
4. If the workload is projected using a relative value recording system that includes all functions (diagnostic work, administration, clerical, media production, etc.), the number of hours for full-time equivalent personnel will be determined directly by projected value.
5. Multiply the projected number of hours required in the computation of steps 3 or 4 by 1.17 to determine the hours that should be budgeted. (Based on projected use of 85% of budgeted hours; see p. 109).
6. Establish simultaneous space use by multiplying the projected number of workers by 0.75.
7. Multiply this value by 100 to establish the minimum net square feet required.

## CHAPTER 6

Developing a Quality Control Program

INTRODUCTION

Systematic methods for detecting and controlling error have become established in almost every branch of technology. Manufacturers have found that indirect surveillance of quality, which depends on consumer response to product deficiencies, leads business to the competition before corrective action can be taken. Because of the captive nature of the consumers of hospital laboratory service, efficient detection of error has sometimes been allowed to fall to a level dependent only on complaints voiced by the medical staff. Most laboratory directors have been conscious of the inefficiency of error detection by this means. The lack of guidelines for an organized approach, combined with a willingness on the part of both clinicians and laboratory workers to accept what they assumed to be infrequent occurrences of error, led to an apathetic attitude toward quality control in most laboratories. Persistent pressure to process more specimens and increase the complexity of analysis within the confines of relatively fixed budgets has also contributed to the neglect of quality control activity.

A change in attitude resulted from an increasing recognition among clinical laboratory professional groups of the need to develop guidelines and conduct educational programs to instruct personnel in the development of quality control procedures. Almost simultaneously, and in cooperation with these efforts, state and federal agencies concerned with laboratory licensure introduced recommendations for standards to evaluate laboratory proficiency. The distribution of unknown cultures has been conducted by health

---

1 Current laboratory manual
   (a) Analytical procedures, dated
   (b) References to sources of methods
   (c) Quality control and standardization criteria
2 Dated records of
   (a) Changes in procedure
   (b) Monitoring including remedial action
3 Staining materials
   (a) Test with control smears
4 Media
   (a) Test each batch before use or concurrently with
      selected cultures
5 Serology
   (a) Positive and negative controls
   (b) Controls of graded reactivity or titer

Figure 6-1 Summary of Public Health Service Regulations effective November 15, 1968, Federal Register (33 F.R. 15297-15303). These were developed for quality control activity in clinical laboratories engaged in interstate commerce.

departments and professional societies for many years in an effort to evaluate and improve the capacity for identifying pathogens. Unfortunately this approach yielded little information about handling routine clinical specimens. It did determine that many laboratory workers could not demonstrate sufficient knowledge or proper use of materials for identifying important and common pathogens, even when they knew they were being tested. In 1968 federal regulations for quality control functions were established in laboratories participating in interstate commerce (1). For the first time procedural criteria, which should provide assurance of a minimum standard of quality performance, were established.

These activities motivated laboratory directors to work toward genuine control activities instead of settling for perfunctory measures that would meet the requirements for licensure. Knowledge of this serious attitude among coworkers and professional colleagues provided the third and most significant source of stimulation to workers in microbiology laboratories. A survey conducted by the author of the quality control practices of 100 bacteriology laboratories in 1969 demonstrated that numerous controls had been introduced, many in a majority of laboratories (Figure 6-2a). As programs were being developed in these laboratories, other laboratory directors complained that they lacked sufficient staff or space to initiate the most primitive form of quality control. Exposure to the extensive surveillance activities of large laboratories only served as a source of frustration to workers performing small volumes of bacteriology who could foresee prohibitive increases in work resulting from the introduction of similar quality control procedures in their own laboratories.

Sources of error may differ in small and large laboratories. A large laboratory may monitor a new batch of a culture medium once at the time it is

Specimens sent to reference lab for confirmation	87%
CAP survey	82%
Standard method susceptibility testing	81%
ASCP check samples	78%
Discard chipped glassware	75%
Monitor anaerobic jars	73%
Monitor hot air sterilizers and autoclaves	72%
Test all media for sterility before use	60%
Maintain stock culture collection	60%
Label all media in tubes and plates	58%
Examine direct Gram stained smears on all specimens	53%
Test antigens against control antisera	50%
Date all tubes and plates when prepared	46%
Blind unknowns	46%
Date all dehydrated media when received	45%
Record maintenance on microscopes	41%
Test reagents with stock cultures	40%
Test antisera against control cultures	40%
Use positive slide for ZN control	38%
Test same media before use with control cultures	35%
Use uninoculated incubated control media for each medium used daily	35%
Date all dehydrated media when opened	30%
Record maintenance schedules for pumps, and other motor driven equipment	22%
Record time and pressure on all batches of media	22%
Compute susceptibility profiles	20%
Test night workers periodically	20%
Monitor detergent use	19%
Monitor humidification pans	17%
Use control strains for susceptibility testing	16%
Monitor flow of air in safety hood	15%
Test all media before use with control cultures	15%

Figure 6-2a Distribution of quality control activities in 100 bacteriology laboratories surveyed in 1969.

Item	Observations	Errors	Percentage
1 Susceptibility test controls	56	23	41%
2 Media	2700	500*	18%
3 Reference lab serology	178	13	7%
4 Reference lab cultures	392	22	5%
5 Labeling, dating	6836	245	4%
6 Controls not recorded	3000	115	4%
7 Equipment	1683	48	4%
8 Controls not run	3000	48	2%
9 Use outdated materials	6836	60	1%
10 Serologic controls out	1523	12	1%
	26,201	1205	4.6%

* Breakdown is given in Figures 6-25 and 6-27.

Figure 6-2b Frequency of detection of errors by surveillance activities during 1973 in Hartford Hospital microbiology laboratory.

prepared and finding it acceptable release it for use. It may be used up within a week or two by personnel who observe all of the types of reactions that may occur on this medium frequently enough to assure proper interpretation. The small laboratory may use this medium once every 2 weeks and store it for 6 or 8 months. They have the additional problem of assuring the consistent performance of the medium and proper interpretation by personnel during that period. This may require that the small laboratory spend a larger proportion of its time on quality control than the larger laboratory.

Some laboratories have gained sufficient experience with quality control to allow relative priorities to be placed on various activities. When quality control activities were introduced and progressively developed in our laboratory, we had to be guided by the identification of *potential* problem areas.

We knew this might lead to some surveillance that would prove unproductive. But without monitoring potential sources of trouble, no one could learn how often error would be detected. Figure 6-2*b* illustrates which activities have detected the highest frequency of error in our laboratory. Similar data has been collected for media surveillance (see Figures 6-23, 6-24, and 6-25). This chapter also describes specific surveillance and control activities that may be introduced in microbiology. In each section *basic* elements that should be given first priority are presented. This is followed by suggestions for expanding activities as part of a *more complete* program. These should not be developed until all first priority activities have been initiated. In some sections recommendations are made for activities that might be undertaken by a *more advanced* program. These obviously could be implemented only after most activities for a *more complete* program had been instituted. It is hoped that this will help to avoid the risk of becoming excessively engaged in specialized activities of low or unknown yield before more basic and productive activities are started. It will also allow a progressive involvement in quality control activities, which can be expanded as resources are made available.

DEVELOPING A PROCEDURE MANUAL (BASIC)

The contents of a laboratory manual were extensively discussed in Chapter 3. Preparation of a manual must be the first step in initiating a quality control program. It should be apparent that surveillance cannot be introduced without standards that define expected performance. Six months to a year of effort is required to complete a procedure manual. Development of other quality control activities may overlap this effort as soon as the procedure manual establishes standards for items to be monitored.

Someone must be assigned to develop an outline and to supervise the development and perhaps the writing of this manual. In a small laboratory this may be the only person who is engaged in bacteriology. In larger laboratories the director may assume this responsibility or delegate it to subordinate personnel. In the latter case individual sections of the manual may be prepared by different people, but someone must maintain organization and editorial consistency, and provide motivation for the completion of the task. This requires the permanent allocation of a specific amount of time to quality control. Following the completion of the manual, part of this time must be applied to periodic surveillance of its content to prevent obsolescence. A major pitfall that we observed in following the evolution of quality control programs has been the development of a manual which becomes obsolete while personnel turn their attention to other aspects of quality control. Therefore, following the production of the procedure manual, the second item of priority is the identification of personnel and an appropriate portion of their time for periodic surveillance of the manual in addition to the development of other quality control activities. When errors are found in the manual they should be documented on some regular report (vide infra) which is reviewed with other problems until they are resolved.

RESPONSIBILITY FOR ADMINISTERING THE PROGRAM (BASIC)

Delegation and distribution of responsibility is not a problem in small laboratories since it is only a question of how much time one person can afford to spend. In larger laboratories, employing two or three persons in microbiology, the need for delegating this responsibility is apparent. Someone must maintain a broad supervisory relationship to quality control activities and be assured that they are being conducted according to an established schedule. Obstacles and errors that are encountered must be documented and reported to this person along with the nature of corrective action that is taken. The actual preparation of the procedure manual and the conduct of subsequently developed quality control procedures can be delegated to a subordinate worker. As the size of the laboratory increases, one has the choice of delegating these responsibilities to one primary quality control technologist or of dispersing them among the laboratory staff.

It is impossible to suggest what proportion of time should be allocated to quality control. The percentage relates inversely to the size of the laboratory. More important, it depends on internal and external pressures and the resulting arrangement of priorities for the use of personnel resources. Large laboratories, including ours, spend 5–10% of man-hours on quality control. We have assisted a small laboratory in the development of a limited quality control program. About 2000 bacteriologic specimens were processed per year. Twenty hours per week were applied to bacteriology. One half hour per day is spent on quality control (13%).

THE SURVEILLANCE SCHEDULE AND THE SURVEILLANCE REPORT (BASIC)

As soon as the responsibility for developing and conducting the quality control program is established a *surveillance schedule* must be developed to list all items subject to surveillance. This must include the frequency of surveillance and the range of acceptable performance. Various types of tables and graphs may be prepared to assist in keeping track of observations. These are illustrated throughout this chapter. The surveillance schedule used in our laboratory, and an example of a surveillance report submitted by personnel to document surveillance activities, appears in Appendix I.

In any quality control program other responsibilities occasionally prevent surveillance from being conducted according to schedule. In a small laboratory one person may be responsible for the program and conduct all of the surveillance. A glance at the records provides a reminder of any activities that have fallen behind. In large laboratories the responsibility may reside with the director or the microbiologist. In this case surveillance may be conducted by a number of workers. Records may be kept wherever they are most convenient to the worker who conducts the surveillance. Under these circumstances omissions or delays in conducting surveillance functions may go unrecognized by the director or microbiologist. We have found that workers who would promptly report an observation of error are loathe to report their inability to conduct surveillance as scheduled because of fear of reprimand. Surveillance effort sinks to a lower priority under the pressure of other duties. Technologists readily accept the need to work overtime to complete diagnostic work but rarely use this means to catch up on incomplete quality control activities.

Insidious discontinuation of one surveillance activity after another may occur because of a natural human tendency to ignore inconspicuous responsibilities, especially when no feedback occurs. Those responsible for the program may be lulled into complacency by the lack or decrease of reports of error, which in reality are a result of decreased surveillance. Periodic reports documenting regular surveillance must be required in addition to those reporting erratic performance. This is conducted in the author's laboratory through a *monthly surveillance report*, an example of which appears in Appendix I. The director should modify the frequency, or eliminate surveillance of items that are of a lower priority than others, if an analysis of work conditions precludes a reasonable opportunity to complete the work on time each month.

This report also provides a means of consolidating observations of erratic performance with corrective action taken and ultimate disposition of the problem. Until the matter is completely resolved it is marked "pending" and is reviewed with each month's report. No matter what the size of the laboratory, this form of documentation is essential. It soon becomes apparent that it is not possible to make complete notations of erratic performance and corrective action on graphs and tables used by workers to record primary surveillance data (see Figure 6-3). Erratic performance may be circled or checked in red pencil, but a separate report should be prepared allowing enough space for a complete description of the matter and its ultimate disposition (see Figures AI-1–10, pp. 216–225). These reports will be anticipated by inspectors from performance evaluation agencies because they signify a thorough and well-documented activity.

INVENTORY OF MATERIALS (BASIC, MORE COMPLETE, AND MORE ADVANCED)

This represents a list of biological and chemical reagents purchased and consumed by the laboratory. The intent is to standardize the unit volume in

(Week Ending)	1/7	1/14	1/21	1/28	2/4	2/11	2/18	2/25	3/3	3/10	3/17	3/24	3/31
Temperatures													
Refrigerators #1 Foster-Bact.	7°	7°	(8.5)	7°	(9°)	8°	(9°)	(8.5)	(12°)	7°	7°	7°	7°
#2 Foster-Bacti	6°	6°	7°	6°	6°	6°	6°	6°	6°	6°	6°	7°	7°
#3 Jewett-Serol.	3.5°	3°	7°	3°	5°	3°	2°	3°	3°	3°	(8.5)	8°	6°
#4 Dillon Lilly-QC	4°	5°	5°	8°	4°	4°	3°	3°	2°	5°	5°	3°	4°
Waterbaths #1 TSA Bact No.4608A	48.8	48.5	48.8	47.5	47	48	48	48	49	47.5	48	48	48
#2 misc Bact No.0264	—	—	—	—	—	—	—	—	—	—	—	—	—
#3 VDRL Serol No.515	56°	56°	top off CrRA Stain 53°	55°	55°	(52° 20H₂O)	(53°)	56°	57°	56°	56°	56°	57
#4 misc Serol No.0964	37°	37°	37°	37°	36°	36°	39°	37°	39°	37°	37°	36°	36
#5 module Bact Heater	(46°) New Range set 46° see change		—	—	—	46°	39°	45	—	(43)	46	46	46
#6 module Bacti Heater	(46°)	46°	—	—	—	(48°)	45°	45	46	46	46	46	46
#7 Elconmp Bact 400/2	(53°)	(58°)	(53)	—	—	(53)	—	55°	—	(60°)	54	55	(52)

Figure 6-3 Common method of recording surveillance. Note that erratic temperatures are circled, but no record is provided of action taken to correct deficiency. Inadequate, brief, and sometimes cryptic notes are written in available space. Attention should be drawn to observations that exceed control limits. A description of the problem, efforts to resolve it, and ultimate disposition should be recorded more completely elsewhere. See Figures 6-9 and the surveillance report in Appendix I (Figure A1-7) for the correct handling of surveillance.

Week Ending	4/9	4/11	4/16	4/18	4/23	4/25	4/30	5/2	5/7	5/9	5/14	5/16	5/21
Incubators Temp. #1 Labline	35°	35°	35°	35°	(34.5°)	35°	35°	36°	35°	36°	36°	38°	35°
#2 Elconap med A-5	35°	35°	35°	36°	36°	35°	35°	35°	36°	(34.5°)	35°	35°	35°
#3 Labline-CO₂	35°	35°	35°	36°	35°	35°	36°	35°	35°	35°	35°	35°	35°
Miscellaneous #1 Fans	of	OK	OK	OK	Rattle- also motor Needed	Rattle- New motor needed	→	→	Rattle	Rattle	Being repaired	Being Repaired	OK
#1 Water	OK	OK	OK	OK	OK	OK	OK	OK	OK	OK	OK	OK	OK
#2 Water	OK	OK	OK	OK	OK	OK	OK	Not in use	→	→	→	→	→
#3 Water	OK	OK	OK	OK	OK	OK	OK	OK	OK	OK	OK	OK	OK
#3 Humidity(%)	64	74	69	70	68	69	68	69	70	68	69	87	68
#3 CO₂ Flow (LPM)	.3	.3	.3	.3	.3	.3	.3	.3	.3	.3	.3	.3	.3
#3 CO₂ tank Pressure	200	900	800	800	700	700	700	650	600	Surge 500 Flow 900	Surge 300 Flow 900	Surge 900 Flow 900	Surge 900 Flow 900
#3 CO₂ Conc(%)	on analyzer	→	→	→	→	→	→	awaiting new gauges	on analyzer	→	→	
Morgue refrig.	47	46	51	47	50	48	46	47	46	46	47	46	46

Figure 6-3 (cont.)

which things are purchased and the conditions and duration of storage. The need for such a system is apparent from a casual inspection of the materials commonly found in microbiology laboratories. Various reagents are frequently stored indefinitely after they have been obtained for a trial of a procedure that was subsequently abandoned. These occupy space and interfere with the proper organization of materials required for conducting established procedures. Certain materials must be maintained for performing tests that are required but infrequently performed. A common discouraging experience in laboratories is to find that such materials have expired or are unsatisfactory when they are needed. The first step in developing an inventory is to eliminate all materials that are not required for any established procedure or active development project.

The first items to be listed in the preparation of a *basic* inventory should be those that are infrequently used and are subject to deterioration with prolonged storage. Before deciding to list such an item the director should consider referring the test to another laboratory, thus allowing the elimi-

	January	February	March	April	May	June
Serology Controls Aso titer	OK	one week Behind	2 controls omitted	OL	OK - one control below accept. ran. New Control made	OK
Brucella	OK	OL	OL	OK	one control above acceptable limit Repeated-Same	OL
Cold Agglut	one control not recorded	OL	one control not recorded	OK	Control consist. above accept. limit. New range set	OL
C.R.P.	One lot nbr. not recorded	OK	two controls not recorded	one control lot nbr. not recorded	ok	one Control not recorded
Leptospira	OK	OK	OK	ok	NOT Run	ok
Monospot	1 lot. nbr. not recorded	3 cont. not recorded	OL	OK	OK	OL
R.A. Latex	8 slide controls Not recorded 1 lot nbr. not recorded	2 controls not rec. 2 lot nbr. not rec.	OK	2 Controls Not Recorded 1 control lot nbr. not recorded	6 control lot nbr. answers not recorded	1 control Not recor.
Typhoid	ok	1 lot nbr not recorded	OL	one antigen lot nbr. not recorded	OL	OL
Thyroglobulin	4 lot nbr. not recorded	4 lot nbr. not recorded	one antigen lot nbr. not recorded	one antigen lot nbr. not recorded	OK	ok
VDRL	OK 1 exceeded range	OK	ok	1 exceeded range	OK	ok
Fluorescent ANF	OK	OL	ok	ok	ok	OK
E. coli	OK	ok	OK	OK	OK	OL
N. Gonorr.	OK	OL	OK	OL	OK	OK
R.A.-ZN.	OK	OK	OK	OK	OL	OL
Strep	OK	OK	OL	OK	OL	OL
Clin. Mic. Benzidine	OL	OL	OL	OL	OL	OL
Urine Control	ok	Not very many spec. put through	4/1 Calculated	OK	ok	7/2 Calcula.

Figure 6-3 (cont.)

nation of reagents used for its performance from the inventory. If materials must be maintained for performing such procedures, they should be purchased in the smallest available quantity. For example, it would be foolish to purchase Fletcher's medium in 1 lb bottles if it is unlikely that any will be prepared for a potential case of Leptospirosis within 1 or 2 years of purchase. Instead, the inventory should specify ¼ lb bottles or smaller packages. It is less desirable to purchase such infrequently used media in prepared form because of the shorter shelf life, but this may be acceptable if the laboratory is unable to prepare its own. Another example might be the storage of Diphtheria antitoxin strips for the performance of an in vitro toxigenicity test. The laboratory director must again determine whether it would be preferable to perform this test in his own laboratory on a suspected isolate or submit the culture to a referral laboratory. If these strips are to be kept on hand, they should be maintained frozen for a maximum of 1 year after which they should be discarded and replaced with new stock.

It will become progressively apparent to the worker developing such an inventory that a substantial number of materials may be required to perform tests that are infrequently requested. The problem of inadequate workloads is reviewed elsewhere in this book. The necessity of establishing an extensive inventory of infrequently used materials may add further impetus to the elimination of these procedures if referral services are available.

The next step in the preparation of a *more complete* inventory is to list all other biologicals and chemical reagents subject to deterioration. High priority items include prepared and dehydrated media, antigens and antisera, antimicrobial disks, and labile reagents purchased in the prepared form for oxidase, indole, and Voges-Proskauer tests. If the biochemical tests are performed with reagents that are prepared by the laboratory from stock chemicals, these may be given a lower priority listing when they possess increased stability.

Most antigens and antisera display expiration dates that are provided by the manufacturer. In the absence such information we have established an arbitrary 1 year expiration date. Expiration dates of 2 years for unopened dehydrated media are conservative. Much of this material has an indefinite shelf life. From a practical point of view, it would seem possible to purchase dehydrated media in small enough quantities to prevent the need for more extended periods of storage. Media that has been opened is subject to deterioration and hardening, especially if humid air has been introduced. Once opened dehydrated media should not be kept more than 6 months. The storage of prepared media is a matter of controversy. It is not possible to determine the age of some of the commercial media that is distributed. Much of it is at least 4 weeks old when received. Testing has demonstrated that prepared media can function normally for months and in some cases for years. Studies conducted by Packer and her associates have shown that most media prepared in the laboratory continue to display satisfactory performance for 20 weeks (2). The media must be bagged, and in most instances refrigerated, to prevent evaporation and deterioration. It is obvious that unbagged media, or media in tubes with other than screw caps, will suffer from evaporation within a week or two of preparation. Recent unpublished observations indicate that blood agar and chocolate agar (including Thayer-Martin, Martin-Lester, and Transgro media) are acceptable for as long as 2 months if they are bagged and refrigerated.

An *advanced* inventory may be established by adding all other relatively stable biological and chemical reagents. The limits and conditions of storage for these materials are less critical, and rather aribtrary criteria have been established in our laboratory. Although it might seem unessential to include these materials in the inventory list, we have found that including all reagents and biologicals allows surveillance to be extended to the inventory of all supplies (Figure 6-4). Those personnel assigned to the surveillance of storage and expiration dates of inventory items simultaneously detect the exhaustion or depletion of supplies, which then are reordered.

PERSONNEL PRACTICES (BASIC)

In both small and large laboratories there are procedures that are infrequently performed by personnel. This is especially true of those who work part-time, evenings and nights, or rotate through other laboratory divisions. As an arbitrary recommendation we believe that a *basic* quality control program should require that any procedure not conducted at least once every 4 weeks be performed under supervision on a periodic basis (e.g., once a month). The need for such tests should be reviewed with the medical staff. If they must be available, but need not be performed on an emergency basis, they should be sent out to a referral laboratory. If the immediate performance of a large variety of infrequently executed tests is considered clinically desirable, both the staff and the administration must support the

NAME __Monospot__   MANUFACTURER __Ortho__

date received	Manufact Lot Nbr	Exp date		HH Lot Nbr	Date in Use	TECH
8-28-72	IM 273	10-30-72		N_1	9-20-72	Hld
"	"	"		N_2	9-30-72	B
10-3-72	IM 276	12-10-72		O_1	10-5-72	HN
"	"	"		O_2	10-12-72	B
10-19-72	IM 275	11-20-72		P_1	10-21-72	CP
"	"	"		P_2	11-1-72	LA
11-3-72	IM 280	1-1-73		Q_1	11-6-72	B
"	"	"		Q_2	11-14-72	LH
"	"	"		Q_3	11-22-72	B
12-5-72	IM 282	1-22-73		R_1	12-6-72	B
"	"	"		R_2	12-13-72	LAK
"	"	"		R_3	12-20-72	B
"	IM 285	2-12-73		S_1	12-28-72	HK
"	"	"		S_2	1/4/73	Lla
"	"	"		S_3	1/9/73	B
1-10-73	IM 287	3-5-73		T_1		
"	"	"		T_2		

Figure 6-4   Record maintained for logging in the date of receipt for biologicals (in this case Monospot® reagents for tests for heterophile antibody). This system assures control of expiration, adequacy of inventory, and sequential use of reagents by lot numbers.

laboratory's need to apply sufficient quality control activity to these procedures, thereby assuring their accurate performance. Such a comprehensive review may prove to all concerned that this service is a luxury that the hospital cannot afford to provide.

We have observed many small laboratories in which numerous procedures are so infrequently conducted that personnel should have little confidence in the reliability of the materials or their ability to properly interpret results. Only professional and institutional pride causes many of these institutions to continue performing these procedures themselves. Other alternatives are discussed in Chapter 5 (see Workloads, p. 110). It is important to present any regular review as an educational measure intended to improve the confidence of the worker, not as an inquisition implying a lack of faith in the workers' ability. It should be conducted when it will not interfere with the regular responsibilities of these personnel. This may be accomplished with workers who cover evening and night shifts by paying them to come in one half hour earlier. Experienced workers should conduct these reviews and may be required to come to work early or stay late. The administration should be aware that this may result in some predictable overtime.

An outline of the questions to be asked and the procedures to be conducted during the review should be prepared. A worksheet used in the author's laboratory for workers on the evening and night shift is displayed in Figure 6-5. The frequency with which the review is conducted and the procedures that are included should be based on the performance of routine work and the results of previous reviews. The individual's knowledge of general laboratory policy should be evaluated. This might include the disposition of specimens submitted in improper containers or when a specific procedure is unavailable. If there is a policy that physicians follow to obtain approval for procedures conducted at odd hours, this should be reviewed. It may be desirable to observe the performance and interpretation of Gram stains. This may be accomplished by observing the staining of smears that were received or prepared during the day but have not been Gram stained. A collection of Gram stained smears of spinal fluid, sputum, or wounds may be established to evaluate interpretation. Various types of specimens that have been submitted for culture may be saved to observe proper planting procedure. Even if there is a small volume of bacteriology, this can be accomplished by using broth for body fluids and slightly moistened swabs for throat and wound cultures. Actual specimens of sputum should be used because it is important to review the criteria for determining the adequacy of specimens for culture and the selection of mucopurulent portions for processing. We have found that a strictly narrative review of these matters fails to uncover many misunderstandings and technical errors. Urine specimens containing abnormal sediments may be saved from the day's work for review of chemical and microscopic analysis. About one drop, or 0.05 cc, of full strength formalin for each 5 cc of urine

Employee *JACK JONES*

Microbiology Quality Control

Evening & Night Shift Personnel Performance Evaluation

Describe specimens for which you are responsible during your shift.

Plant all Bacteriology to 10:30
Do urinalyses from ER to 11 PM, from
floors until 9 PM

Describe tests which you may perform only after approval.

Pregnancy tests

	For Evaluation		Satisfactory	See SR
Planting:	Fluids ( )	Eye ( )		
	Wound (✓)	Ear ( )		
	Blood (✓)	Urine ( )		
	CSF ( )	Sputum(✓)		
	Feces ( )			
	Genitalia (✓)			
	Throat ( )			
	Tissue ( )			
	Other *anaerobic Sputum*(✓)			
Choice of Media:			( )	(✓)
Planting Technique:			(✓)	( )
Proper Annotation (date, initials, etc.):			( )	(✓)
Anaerobic, capneic incubation :			( )	(✓)

Figure 6-5 Worksheet for performing an evaluation of personnel who work evening or night shifts. The supervisor selects procedures that are to be reviewed. Evaluation is conducted by the assistant supervisor, who works the late shift when such evaluations are conducted. Collection of Gram stains is used to evaluate interpretive skills. See Figure AI-2, page 217, for evaluation of performance in monthly surveillance report (SR).

-2-

Gram Stain:	For Evaluation	Satisfactory	See SR
Performance	(✓)	(✓)	( )
Interpretation	(✓)		

Unknown

16
Sput

1. RBC   0
NEUT.   0
LYMPH. 0
BACT.   2+

Gram pos cocci 2+ ( )

Gram neg rods 1+

Q3

(✓)

27
CSF

2. RCB   0
NEUT.   2+
LYMPH. 0
BACT.   3+

Pleomorphic Gram (✓)
neg coccobacilli

( )

31
Wound

3. RBC   1+
NEUT.   3+
LYMPH. 1+
BACT.   2+

Gram pos rods (✓)

( )

35
CSF

4. RBC   0
NEUT.   3+
LYMPH. 0
BACT.   3+

Gram pos cocci (✓)

( )

Urinalysis:		(✓)	( )
CSF Cell Count:		(✓)	( )
Pregnancy Test:		(✓)	( )

New Procedures or Changes in Location of Materials: (✓) None

Record any deficiencies on Surveillance Report along with employee's comments.

Next Review Suggested: ( ) 1 month   (✓) 3 months   ( ) 6 months

Evaluation Conducted by _Ann Smith_   Date: _12/5/72_

Figure 6-5 (cont.)

preserves cells and casts for 18–24 hours and does not interfere with chemical tests, including glucose determination by glucose oxidase.

The *surveillance schedule* should indicate the frequency with which such reviews are conducted and the *surveillance report* should show whether they are conducted and whether deficiencies were observed. Corrective action might include separately scheduled training exercises, reading, or a repeat review. Consistently inadequate performance might result in a recommendation for termination. Reports of consistently good performance would be helpful in supporting requests for advancement. Good performance should also cause a decrease in the frequency of scheduled reviews.

USE OF THE REFERENCE LABORATORY (BASIC)

Most laboratories make incomplete use of results returned from other laboratories on specimens that have been submitted for their examination. In some cases reference laboratories are only used when required by law. For example, in Connecticut *Salmonellae* and *Shigellae* must be submitted for confirmation of speciation and serotyping. Many laboratories also submit atypical isolates for speciation or confirmation of speciation. As a *basic* element of a quality control program some arrangement should be established with a reference laboratory for periodic examination of problem isolates. The reference laboratory may be a state health department laboratory or a major medical center laboratory. The use made of such reports depends on the extent of the data returned. Some reference laboratories indicate only the species and do not provide substantiating biochemical and serologic observations. Because of the intense interest of most health departments in performance evaluation and quality control, pressure should be exerted by laboratory directors for provision of such data when health department laboratories are used for reference purposes.

A system should be developed within the laboratory to maintain a viable subculture of any isolate submitted to a reference laboratory. When the results are returned these should be systematically compared with the speciation and criteria originally observed (Figure 6-6). When discrepancies are observed tests should be repeated. If discrepancies continue to occur, these should be pursued until they are resolved. They may result from differences in media, reagents, or criteria for interpretation. Figure 6-7 demonstrates the types of discrepancies that have been observed through the use of such a system in the author's laboratory. The most common discrepancies were: (1) mixed cultures; (2) premature interpretation of tests involving carbohydrate utilization; (3) failure to perform flagella stains; (4) incorrect interpretation of oxidase tests; (5) false positive agglutination tests for enteropathogenic *Escherichia coli*. A rigorous attempt to resolve discrepancies reveals many other errors in performance and interpretation. Not infrequently the problem is found to lie in the reference laboratory. A good rapport should be established with the director of the reference laboratory to allow an open and informal approach to the resolution of persistent discrepancies. If these are due to differences in media or serologic reagents, consideration should be given to standardizing on the materials used in the reference laboratory. Similarly, criteria for interpretation that depend on color or time for developing certain reactions may require restandardization.

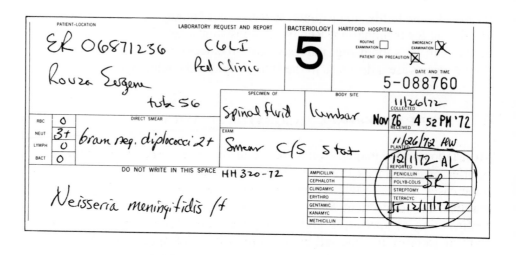

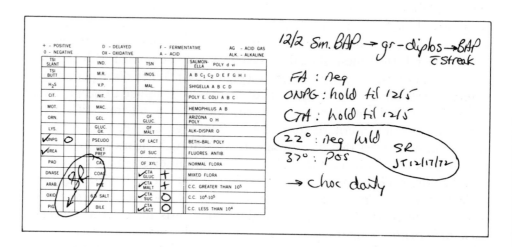

Figure 6-6 Report slips from cultures submitted to reference labs are copied and displayed alongside reference laboratory report. This facilitates the comparison of results. Note delays and discrepancy in growth at 22°C. These are recorded in surveillance report (see Appendix, Figure AI-3, p. 218).

CONNECTICUT STATE DEPARTMENT OF HEALTH

TEL. 566-2536

LABORATORY DIVISION

10 Clinton Street

P. O. BOX 1689, HARTFORD, CONN. 06101

REPORT ON CULTURES FOR CLASSIFICATION

Specimen No. HH320-73 Date received   Dec. 2, 1972   Date reported   Dec. 12, 1972

Report of
examination of   *Spinal Fluid*

For   *Neisseria speciation*

Sender's name and address	Patient's name and address
RAYMOND C. BARTLETT, M. D. HARTFORD HOSPITAL 80 SEYMOUR STREET HARTFORD, CONNECTICUT 06115	*Rouza, Eugene* *53 State St* *Hartford, Conn* AGE:

This culture is classified as:

    Neisseria subflava

BIOCHEMICAL REACTIONS AFTER			DAYS INCUBATION			MORPHOLOGY, STAINING, ETC.
Glucose	A *		Sorbitol			gram negative diplococci
Lactose	—		Adonitol			Motility negative
Sucrose	—		Citrate			Colony Type
Salicin			Purple milk			MacConkey Agar:
Maltose	A *		Urea			No growth
~~Mannitol~~ *Fructose*	— *		V. P.			
Rhamnose			Indole			Blood Agar:
Arabinose			Oxidase			non-hemolytic
Raffinose			Gelatine			SEROLOGICAL REACTIONS
Inositol			Nitrate			Neisseria meningitidis antisera
Dulcitol			H₂S - PbAc strip			groups A-D negativve
Xylose			Starch			Slaterus
Triple	Butt		Glycogen			types X-Z negative
Sugar Iron	Slant		Galactose			
Agar	H₂S		Catalase			

A=Acid   G=Gas   AG=Acid and Gas.   Ability to form gas absent unless recorded under Glucose.

Remarks:

        *Biochemical reactions are in <u>Neisseria</u> base sugars.

        Growth at 22 C: positive

AP ....

Form OL-136 (12-70) 5M   Director

Figure 6-6 (cont.)

The *surveillance schedule* should state that this comparative process is conducted on all isolates that are sent out and that resolution of discrepancies will occur. As with any surveillance measure someone must monitor each isolate regularly to assure that this is being done. If unresolved discrepancies are found, this should be reported to the director in the *surveillance report* with proposed action for final resolution of the problem.

Bacteriology	Error	Number	Explanation
Morphology			
Gram stain	FP	1	Overdecolorization
Motility	O	2	Omitted
Flagella	O	7	Omitted
	RE	1	Reference lab omitted. Disagreement on morphology
	UD	1	Unresolved
Biochemical			
Catalase	UD	1	Unresolved
Carbohydrate	FN	15	Premature interpretation
Fermentation	FP	13	Contamination
	UD	8	Unresolved
Urea hydrolysis	FP	3	Contamination
	UD	3	Unresolved
Gelatin liquefaction	FP	1	Contamination
	FN	1	Insufficient inoculum
	UD	2	Unresolved
Nitrate reduction	FP	4	Contamination
	UD	1	Unresolved
	FN	1	Insufficient growth
Indole	FP	2	Contamination
	FN	1	Delayed reaction (6 days)
		3	Insufficient inoculum
Voges Proskauer	FN	2	Premature analysis
	UD	1	Unresolved
Citrate utilization	UD	1	Unresolved
Methyl red	FP	1	Contamination
H_2S (lead acetate)	FN	1	Premature interpretation
	UD	3	Unresolved
H_2S (TSI)	FP	1	Contamination
	O	1	Omitted
	UD	1	Unresolved
Ornithine	FN	1	Insufficient growth
Lysine decarboxylase	O	1	Omitted
	FP	3	Insufficient acid produced in Falkow medium
	UD	1	Unresolved
Oxidase	FN	1	Reagents inactive
	UD	1	Unresolved
	FP	6	Delayed interpretation and oxidized paper strips
	FN	1	Incorrect interpretation
Phenylalanine deaminase	FN	1	Phenylalanine omitted in media
Gluconate oxidation	FN	1	Use of Ca^{++} instead of K^+ gluconate
45° tolerance	O	3	Omitted
TSI	FN	1	Insufficient growth

Figure 6-7 Resolution of discrepancies between results obtained in the author's laboratory and those obtained on the same 217 isolates in a reference laboratory.
FP = false positive observation, confirmed by reexamination of cultures.
FN = false negative observation, confirmed by reexamination of cultures.
O = omitted when observation would have been useful in characterizing culture.
UD = unresolved discrepancy in spite of reexamination of cultures by both laboratories, probably due to differences in acceptable techniques used by each. RE = reference lab error.

140

Figure 6-7 (cont.)

Serological			
Enteropathogenic *E. coli*	FP	5	Bile salts in media
	RE	4	False negative in reference laboratory
	UD	1	Unresolved
H. influenza	FN	3	Inavid antiserum
E. coli (alkalescens-dispar)	FN	3	Blocking, failure to heat
	O	1	Omitted
Shigella	FN	1	Rough when typed

As a portion of a *basic* quality control program, sera may be submitted to reference laboratories to compare the results of tests for antibodies. Figure 6-8 demonstrates the outcome of a comparison of the VDRL titer on all sera found to be reactive in the author's laboratory with results returned from a reference laboratory where the test was repeated on the same specimen. This might seem unessential in view of the periodic examinations for certification and use of highly standardized control sera provided by state health department laboratories. It has allowed us to detect periodic deviations in the interpretive criteria of various personnel. It also provides an example of the type of data that could be collected for any serologic test where standardization between two laboratories is desired. It is likely that most other serologic tests would not demonstrate as good a correlation unless identical sources of antigens and antisera were used. This reflects the problem of the lack of standardization of commercial serological reagents (see Chapter 3, p. 65).

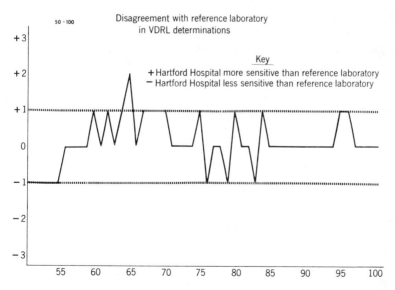

Figure 6-8 Disagreement in twofold dilutions for VDRL performed on reactive sera by the author's laboratory and a reference laboratory on the same specimen. The procedure helps to prevent insidious changes in standards that occur in spite of the daily use of control sera.

EQUIPMENT (BASIC AND MORE COMPLETE)

Regular monitoring of laboratory equipment is easily established and should be considered a *basic* element of a quality control program. First priority should be given to incubators, water baths, refrigerators, and freezers. Temperature may be monitored by chart recorders, but this will cost more than $300 for each instrument. For alarms that ring if upper and lower established limits are exceeded, more than $100 is required.

In some laboratories blood bank refrigerators are monitored around the clock by connecting "hi-low" sensors to alarms in the security office. One commercial organization has made a business of monitoring equipment in numerous industrial and research laboratories through permanent lines leading to a monitoring center. We do not know of any microbiology laboratories that have used such a system. An inventory of a small refrigerator in our laboratory revealed its content to be worth in excess of $200. On one occasion we discarded most of this material because of deterioration due to equipment failure that was not detected until the thermometers were checked. It seems justifiable and desirable to spend enough money to obtain monitors that will alert someone immediately in case of power or equipment failure.

If greater economy is dictated, the commonly available high and low temperature thermometers, which contain metal slugs in the two capillary channels, may be installed. These may be reset with a magnet. The position of the slugs establishes the maximum and minimum temperatures reached since resetting. Daily examination of the thermometers is the least expensive and least effective approach (Figure 6-9). Incubators are often provided with built-in thermometers. A further disadvantage is that such thermometers reflect changes in temperature immediately following the opening of the door. Thermometers placed in a flask of water are not affected by sudden changes

Week Ending	10/14	10/21	10/28	11/4	11/11	11/18	11/25	12/2	12/9	12/16	12/23	12/30
Refrigerators												
MB 4338-Foster 4	4°	4°	5°	4°	7°	4°	3°	4°	6°	5°	5°	5°
MB 4339-Foster 2	SR 10/18 7°	5°	5°	5°	SR 11/13 7°	6°	5°	4°	SR 12/14 7°	5°	4°	4°
MB 4340-Foster 6	4°	4°	4°	5°	4°	4°	4°	4°	5°	4°	3°	4°

Figure 6-9 Surveillance record of weekly refrigerator temperatures. After each week that a temperature of 7°C was recorded, the temperature exceeded upper limits and the alarms sounded. The notation "SR" indicates that a complete description of problem can be found in the surveillance report (See Figure AI-7, p. 222). Note that the alarms sounded on a day other than the routine weekly temperature check. The latter may be considered a check on the calibration of the alarms.

in temperatures, but provide an index of changes taking place over several hours. Liquids, such as propylene glycol, may be used in deep freezes. Thermometers that are shipped with waterbaths may show error of 1 or 2°C. All thermometers should be calibrated against a National Bureau of Standards thermometer, if one is available in the laboratory. Otherwise the manufacturer should provide assurance that the thermometer meets NBS standards within 0.5°C. General maintenance of refrigerators and freezers should include defrosting and cleaning. These procedures are not carried out in some laboratories unless a specific schedule is established. Backup equipment must be available to maintain proper storage conditions for defrosting. Improper circulation of air in both incubators and refrigerators may cause a marked variation in temperatures in various parts of the device. New equipment should be tested for such irregularities. With increasing use, resulting in obstructed air flow from overloading, repeated measurements should be taken. This is helpful in providing justification for additinal equipment.

For general laboratory purposes incubators should be maintained at 35,± 1°C, waterbaths at 37 ± 0.5°C, or other temperatures with appropriate ranges for other applications; freezers suitable for materials that need only to be kept below freezing at −5 to −1°C; deep freezes at −20 ± 5°C; and ultra-deep freezes at −50 ± 10°C. Humidification is commonly neglected in incubators. Adequate amounts of water in humidification pans should be monitored several times a week.

Routine maintenance of other electrical and mechanical devices should be reviewed and a schedule established with a representative from the engineering or maintenance department. This should include ventilating equipment and filters. Although laboratory personnel may not conduct such maintenance, they may establish a surveillance procedure to verify that the maintenance *has* been conducted on schedule. Failure of fans producing air circulation in incubators has been a common problem in our laboratory. Initially this required shutting down the incubator while replacement motors were obtained. In recent years replacement motors and other parts subject to failure have been kept in stock for immediate installation in any equipment that requires continuous operation. Backup refrigerators and freezers are continuously available in case failure or routine maintenance requires removal of materials.

A *basic* equipment surveillance program includes monitoring autoclaves and hot air ovens used for sterilization. Hot air ovens should operate between 155 and 165°C. Adequacy of sterilization should be further tested by including spore strips inside the largest mass of material inserted in the oven. In general the minimum length of hot air sterilization should be 1 hour.

A temperature of 121°C should be maintained at the exhaust valve of autoclaves. This requires 15 lb of pressure at sea level. The length of time required to achieve sterilization depends on the volume of liquid in the containers and the number of bacteria in the liquid being processed. Once the fluid has reached 121°C, 12–15 minutes of heating will assure sterility. The adequacy of the length of time may be tested by placing spore strips in the center of dry packages. If liquids are being sterilized, spore solution ampules should be placed in the largest vessel. Adequate sterilization is not established by placing such strips or ampules on the shelf of an autoclave. Unperforated pans should never be used because these trap air and prevent exposure to steam, resulting in incomplete sterilization. Excessive wrapping or tightly capped vessels also interfere with sterilization. Time-temperature recorders should be used and someone should be responsible for monitoring each cycle to establish that adequate time at the minimum temperature was applied to sterilize each load.

Unique sterilization problems associated with the preparation of media are also discussed in this chapter (vide infra). In general it may be said that media require a shorter exposure for sterilization than cultures or other contaminated materials. This is supported by the thermal death curve, which expresses the exponential rate at which bacteria are killed at a sterilizing temperature. An exposure sufficient to sterilize media may be insufficient to sterilize an ampule containing 10^8 spores per milliliter. It would be a mistake to require that media be exposed for a time sufficiently long to sterilize a test suspension of spores.

If specimens and cultures containing mycobacteria or fungi other than strictly opportunistic species are handled, a safety cabinet must be provided. The grinding of tissues should also be performed in such a cabinet. The simplest cabinets represent hoods that are exhausted into a ventilation system or out of a window. A velocity of 50 ft per minute must be maintained through the opening of such a hood. This may be measured with a flow meter, which is commonly used for monitoring air conditioning equipment. Most large institutions possess these in the maintenance department. Although simple hoods and exhaust systems are better than nothing, there is an increasing opinion that hazardous microbiologic materials should be handled in hoods containing air incinerators or ultrafilters that prevent the discharge of hazardous contamination into ductwork or the atmosphere. The handling of lyophilized cultures or pathogens known to represent an extreme laboratory hazard should be conducted only in such a cabinet. The same minimum face velocity should be provided. In addition the drop in pressure across the filter should be monitored. A difference of 10–15 mm of water should be obtained. Any decrease suggests potentially hazardous leaks around the filter. An increase in pressure signifies the need for replacement of the filter. This will probably be associated with a decrease in the face velocity.

The monitoring of air flow configurations within the very useful new laminar flow safety cabinets should not be conducted by clinical laboratory workers. Manufacturers of these devices claim that filters do not require replacement for years and that air flow patterns remain unchanged. We have insisted that a contract for annual testing of these units be established at the time of purchase. Industrial consultants are available to perform this because there is a demand for such monitoring in clean room applications. Smoke pencils and devices capable of measuring low concentrations of airborne particulate matter are required. As long as the face velocity is maintained at 50 ft per minute, the safety of personnel can be assured. Other alterations in internal air configurations only result in potential contamination of the material. The highest priority is obviously the protection of personnel.

In a *basic* quality control program the monitoring of anaerobic jars should be conducted each time they are used with methylene blue or similar Eh indicators. Optionally, a culture of an anaerobe, such as *Clostridium novyii,* that requires an Eh below -100 mv should be tested. Palladium chloride catalysts should be removed periodically and regenerated by heating from 155 to 165°C in a hot air oven for 1 hour. Adherence to these measures should be monitored. If more strictly anaerobic systems are in use, control cultures that require the lowest Eh expected of the system for growth should be provided.

Using chipped or broken glassware represents false economy and a hazard to laboratory workers. Periodic inspection of the glassware in use should be conducted to control this problem. Use of the proper amounts of detergent by those who wash the glassware is another problem. Periodic unobtrusive observation should be conducted to establish whether proper amounts of detergent are being used. Excess residues cause error in serologic procedures and introduce pH variations in solutions. Deionized or distilled water, which meets the more critical standards of chemical analysis, is satisfactory for microbiology. Extremely acid water may produce errors in the pH of media and other solutions. Evidence of residual detergent may be detected by measuring the pH of water before and after it is used for rinsing suspect pieces of glassware. Another simple technique is the addition of a drop of bromcresol purple indicator to a container that has been filled with deionized water. Significant residue produces a distinct violet color.

Most laboratories that possess capneic incubators do not monitor them. In a *more complete* quality control program this may be performed by trapping gas in either a syringe or a balloon and submitting the sample to a pulmonary medicine laboratory experienced in measuring CO_2 in expired air. The effects of frequently opening and closing the door should be studied. Devices that contain automatic surging provide more rapid restitution of CO_2 concentration, but they may also overcompensate. Concentrations of CO_2 that exceed 10 or 15% produce a decrease in the pH of media because of the formation of carbonic acid. Concentrations in the range of 4–10% provide sufficient stimulation for capnophilic bacteria. The most elegant way to monitor CO_2 concentrations is the use of an infrared recording spectrophotometer. Other devices are commercially available but their calibration should be tested with known standard gas mixtures before they are purchased. There is great variation in the reliability of such equipment. Candle jars are very useful for isolating microaerophiles. We have observed oxygen concentrations in the range of 14–16% with CO_2 concentrations between 3 and 6%.

Periodic maintenance should be provided for microscopes. This includes complete cleaning and repair. A log should be kept of work conducted on each microscope together with any complaints from personnel about the performance of the equipment. Such documentation is of great value when replacement requires justification. In a *more advanced* program glassware should be checked for calibration by selecting random pipettes from each shipment. Standard methods for calibrating laboratory glassware should be used. In practice we have found that serological pipettes used in microbiology consistently meet expected tolerance limits when purchased from reputable major suppliers.

DIFFUSION (BAUER-KIRBY) METHOD OF ANTIMICROBIAL SUSCEPTIBILITY TESTING (BASIC, MORE COMPLETE, AND MORE ADVANCED)

In this section attention is focused on the disk diffusion test of Bauer and his associates (3). Other disk diffusion methods are not considered sufficiently well standardized to allow the application of useful and specific control measures. Certain modifications of the method of Bauer et al. are acceptable because they produce insignificantly different results. These include the agar overlay method of Barry and the use of 100 mm plates instead of 150 mm plates, provided that disks are placed no closer than 12.5 mm to the edge of the plate. This may be accomplished with a dispenser (Bioquest 60456). Photometric equilibration of inoculum density produces no advantage over visual equilibration. Other modifications of Bauer's method include the use of a powdered glass standard in place of barium sulfate and the interpretation of zone diameters by using concentric targets instead of measurement with calipers (4–6).

Other common modifications produce detectable variations. These include the use of media other than Mueller-Hinton with or without chocolatized blood, random inoculum densities not standardized in the range of 10^8 colony forming units per milliliter, the inspection of zones with transmitted light instead of reflected light, the use of magnification for inspecting zones and the use of interpretive criteria and disks with content other than those established by Bauer et al. The latter methods have been subject to some accepted modifications by subsequent publications and recommendations of NCCLS. These are included in package inserts with antimicrobial disks under the authority and approval of the FDA.

Cultures should be obtained of the original Seattle control strains of *Staphylococcus aureus* ATCC 25923 and *Escherichia coli* ATCC 25922 for *basic* quality control of this test. These may be propagated for 6 months on a nutrient agar slant with storage in a refrigerator. Subcultures should be prepared every 2 weeks. For storage of as long as 2 years, these cultures may be kept frozen in 50% fetal calf's serum at $-20°C$, in liquid nitrogen or lyophilized. Suitable steps should be taken to determine whether contamination or alteration in susceptibility has occurred. With the above methods and durations of storage, the author and other workers have observed no significant change in zone diameters. Isolated colonies should be picked up in the same manner as in the standard procedure. This should be conducted several times a week and the observed zone diameters should be recorded.

In 1970 the FDA conducted a survey of variability in the performance of this test with the use of the Seattle control strains in a number of well-known clinical microbiology laboratories performing the method of Bauer et al. There was a wider variability among laboratories than within laboratories, a phenomenon observed with many analytical procedures. The mean was considered an estimate of "true value" for zone diameters of the control cultures. The FDA established the acceptable variability for a single determination by computing the half interval (to nonstatisticians, about $\pm 1\frac{1}{2}$ standard deviations). This range has been included in the package inserts of all disks. When a single control value exceeds this range it usually turns out to be random variability. There is significant risk, however, that it represents a systematic variable that may cause the reporting of erroneous results. For each drug being tested zone diameters obtained with the Seattle control cultures should be plotted graphically or recorded in a table. Values that exceed the FDA range for accuracy should be circled. If a second consecutive test shows the same variability, an investigation of potential sources should be conducted.

Records should be available to establish any changes in the source of media, disks, or turbidity standard that have occurred coincident with the appearance of erroneous results. The common practice of exhausting the supply of materials previously in use before switching to new batches precludes any comparison that might reveal the source of error when new batches are used. As a general rule, whenever the end of a supply of media or disks of one lot number is approached, a new lot number should be introduced. This not only allows comparison with a possibly defective batch but also provides a temporary source of materials known to produce acceptable results until lots that will produce correct results can be obtained and tested. For these reasons it is best to obtain stocks of media and disks with the same lot number for as long as can be arranged with the supplier. Suppliers often ship random lot numbers if this is not specified. These conditions apply to both commercially prepared and dehydrated media.

Investigation of the causes of a series of erroneous control values in the disk test commonly fails to establish a source. Results often return to acceptable values for no apparent reason. The pH should be rechecked to establish agreement with the value 7.3 ± 1, recommended by Bauer et al. (Bottle labels sometimes indicate other pH values.) The procedure for making correct pH measurements and correcting subsequent batches is discussed on page 166. Alkaline media increase zone diameters for erythromycin and aminoglycosides (kanamycin, neomycin, streptomycin, and gentamicin) and decrease zones for novobiocin, oxacillin, and tetracycline. The reverse is true for acid media. Bacitracin, chloramphenicol, polymyxins, and penicillin are not significantly affected.

It would be desirable to require suppliers to test both dehydrated and prepared media for their ability to produce acceptable zone diameters with the control strains. In the future, government controls may require this of manufacturers. Progress is being made toward developing a completely synthetic defined medium. This will eliminate uncontrolled variables, such as increases in magnesium and calcium concentration, that decrease the activity of tetracyclines and aminoglycosides.

Disk potency may have decreased if zone diameters are erroneously small. Storage conditions should be checked. Semisynthetic penicillins should be kept frozen, others refrigerated, and all dessicated. Purchasing can be controlled to provide shipment of the same lot number. If laboratory workers suspect a bad batch of disks from a supplier, the FDA will test them provided they are shipped to them in a package containing dry ice and with a covering letter. A visit to the local distributor may disclose how long and at what temperature their supply of disks is stored. Most do not keep any disks frozen.

The turbidity standard should be checked for optical density or replaced. Evaporation causes heavy inocula and small zones. Barium sulfate settles out and adheres to glass. It should be resuspended by vortexing each time it is used. Otherwise, there is no evidence that deterioration or decrease in optical density occurs. We found solutions that were used once a week to be stable for 6 months. A variety of storage conditions had no effect on stability; some workers recommend refrigeration.

Control strains may become contaminated. Although they have proved stable with many storage systems, consistent changes in zone diameters observed after more than 6 months of consecutive transfer should signal a need for fresh cultures from a reliable source, such as the American Type Culture Collection, or a local reliable reference laboratory. Other sources of consistent deviation may include: insufficient or excessive rolling out of inoculum before removal of swabs from the tube of inoculum, uneven distribution of inoculum on plates; placement of disk centers closer than 12.5 mm to the edge of the plate or 30 mm to other disks centers; use of wet plates; improper weighing of media or measurement of water; incomplete solution during mixing; uneven or improper thickness of agar in plates; excess drying of plates; a delay of more than 15 minutes in placement of

	Approximate Standard Deviation
1 Inoculum density	0.5–1.0 mm
2 Growth phase	0.5–1.0 mm
3 Disk content	0.5 mm
4 Agar depth	0.5 mm
5 pH and ionic content	Variable
6 Glucose	Variable
7 Water content	Variable
8 Medium composition	1–2 mm
9 Duration of incubation	Variable
10 Zone size measurement	1–2 mm

95% limits of variability = 3 × mean standard deviation = ±3 mm

Figure 6-10 Major sources of variability in disk antimicrobial susceptibility test of Bauer et al. Standard deviations shown are approximate irreducible minimum values achievable through maximum control of variability. Ten variables, each with a standard deviation equal to about 1 mm, yield a net variability of ±3 mm at the 0.95 level of probability. This is comparable to the range of variability actually observed in proficient laboratories.

disks on plates following inoculation; and a delay of more than an additional 15 minutes in placing plates in an incubator (excessive stacking or packing delays the arrival of medium at 35–37°C).

Improper interpretation of zone diameters is a common source of error. Measurement should be conducted using direct illumination against a dark background. Zone edges may appear indistinct and yield smaller measurements if magnification or transmitted light is used. A common pitfall is the performance of the test and the measurement of zone diameters for quality control by an experienced and proficient worker. This may establish that materials are performing correctly but gives no assurance that proper interpretive criteria are being used by all personnel. Review of all sources of variability in this procedure suggests that there may be an irreducible minimum of ±2 to 3 mm (see Figure 6-10).

A *more complete* program may make use of calculations of precision and accuracy that are based on a series of zone diameter values instead of individual measurements. The analysis of precision considers the variance required to produce a significant risk that a true zone diameter falling on the resistant edge of the indeterminate (or intermediate) zone will fall on the susceptible (or sensitive) edge or the converse. Such an error would result in reporting a resistant isolate susceptible or vice versa. The amount of variance that can be allowed depends on the width of the indeterminate zone. If the standard deviation is one half the width of the indeterminate zone, there is a 2% risk that such an error in reporting will occur. This may be called the *maximum standard deviation* in terms of acceptability.

An approach to statistical analysis of precision and accuracy, based on values obtained from five independent samples, was developed by Thomas Gavan, M.D., director of the Department of Microbiology at the Cleveland Clinic (7). Columns labeled "precision control" in Figure 6-11 display values derived by Gavan for the maximum and average differences that should be acceptable for the variation between the highest and lowest of the five zone diameters that are observed. In actual practice precision control has not proved to be a problem. Average standard deviations for precision in selected laboratories have ranged from 0.5 to 1.5 mm (Figure 6-12). Observation of variance in precision exceeding the ranges proposed by Gavan is uncommon and should cause an immediate investigation of sources of inconsistency.

Accuracy is measured by comparing observations with the best estimate of "true value" which, at the present time, is the mean of the results obtained by the FDA. These values are provided in Figure 6-11. Agreement with a "true value" with 99% probability is determined by computing the mean and standard deviation of a series of independent observations. The mean should not exceed the "true value" by more than $\pm 3 \times$ standard deviation/$\sqrt{n}$, where n is the number of observations. An infinite number of observations must produce a mean exactly the same as the "true value." Decreasing numbers of observations allow a larger deviation without disproving the null hypothesis that the observed mean is insignificantly different from the "true value." If this formula is solved for one sample, using maximum standard deviations based on one half the width of the indeterminate zone, a range will be obtained nearly identical to that proposed by the FDA for single values. Figure 6-11 shows the limits over which the mean of five independent values may range and not significantly differ from the "true mean" at the 99% level of probability. Means exceeding this range are commonly observed in laboratories exercising strict controls over performance of this test. Figure 6-15 illustrates results that exceeded acceptable control criteria for accuracy in our laboratory over a 6 month period. Use of the tables developed by Gavan for five independent observations requires no statistical computations other than calculating a mean and should be convenient for any laboratory. Unacceptable results should be evaluated as described on page 147.

There has been some criticism of developing and applying such elegant statistical criteria to the performance of this procedure. Claims that Bauer's method is too qualitative to allow for such treatment are not substantiated by the high degree of precision and accuracy that has been observed in proficient laboratories. Disagreement among laboratories may be the result of variance in media composition, disks, and interpretation of zone diameters.

Simultaneous variance in precision and accuracy summate to increase the risk of an erroneous result. If the observed standard deviation for precision is maximum (one half the width of the indeterminate zone), any variance in accuracy increases the risk of an erroneous result by more than 2%. If the

| Antimicrobic Agent | Disk Content | Escherichia coli (ATCC 25922) | | | | Staphylococcus aureus (ATCC 25923) | | | |
		FDA Mean	Accuracy Control Zone Diameter (mm) Mean of five values	Precision Control Range of five values Maximum	Average	FDA Mean	Accuracy Control Zone Diameter (mm) Mean of five values	Precision Control Range of five values Maximum	Average
Ampicillin	10 mcg	17.5	15.8–19.2	5	2.9		25.8–33.2	11	6.4
Penicillin	10 units		—	—	—	31.5	27.8–35.2	11	6.4
Methicillin	5 mcg			—	—	19.9	17.8–21.2	5	2.9
Cephalothin	30 mcg	20.6	18.8–22.2	5	2.9	31.0	27.0–35.0	12	7.0
Chloramphenicol	30 mcg	24.2	22.0–26.0	6	3.5	22.7	20.2–24.8	7	4.1
Tetraclycline	30 mcg	21.2	19.2–23.0	7	4.1	23.8	20.5–26.5	9	5.2
Erythromycin	15 mcg	11.0	9.0–13.0	6	3.5	26.2	23.3–28.7	8	4.7
Polymyxin	300 units	14.4	12.7–15.3	4	2.3			—	
Kanamycin	30 mcg	21.3	18.3–23.7	8	4.7	22.6	20.2–24.8	7	4.1
Neomycin	30 mcg	20.0	18.0–22.0	6	3.5	—	19.3–24.7	8	4.7
Streptomycin	10 mcg	16.3	13.3–18.7	8	4.7	18.0	15.3–20.7	8	4.7
Gentamicin	10 mcg	22.5	20.2–24.8	7	4.1	—	20.3–25.7	8	4.7

Figure 6-11 Data used to compute the precision and accuracy of the results in five separate tests of control cultures using the disk anti-microbial susceptibility test of Bauer et al (after Gavan).

		Theoretical Maximum Standard Deviations			Observed Standard Deviations									
					Staphylococcus aureus (ATCC 25922)					Escherichia coli (ATCC 25923)				
	I Zone Width	Probability Level			A	B	C	D	E	A	B	C	D	E
		0.01	0.001	0.0001										
Ampicillin {Gram negative	3	1.3	1.0	0.8						1.9	1.3	1.4	1.0	1.2
{Staphylococcus	9	3.9	2.9	2.4	2.2			1.4	2.2					
Cephalothin	4	1.7	1.3	1.1	2.2	1.2	1.4	1.0	2.0	1.3	0.7	1.3	1.3	1.3
Chloramphenicol	6	2.6	1.9	1.6	1.6	1.1	1.7			1.2	0.8	1.1	0.9	
Erythromycin	5	2.2	1.6	1.4	1.5	1.2	1.3	1.0	1.5					
Gentamicin	—	—	—	—									0.5	
Kanamycin	5	2.2	1.6	1.4	1.3		1.5	1.0		1.1	0.9	0.9	0.9	1.3
Methicillin	5	2.2	1.6	1.4	1.6	0.9	1.4	1.0	1.3					
Neomycin	5	2.2	1.6	1.4			0.9					2.1		
Penicillin (Staphylococcus)	9	3.9	2.9	2.4	1.6	1.3	1.1	1.1	1.5					
Streptomycin	4	1.7	1.3	1.1	1.3		1.3	1.0		1.8	0.9	1.4	0.7	
Tetracycline	5	2.2	1.6	1.4	1.6	0.8	1.8			1.2	0.9	1.7	1.3	1.5
Polymyxin B.	4	1.7	1.3	1.1						1.4			0.6	0.7
Colistin	3	1.3	1.0	0.8								0.7		
Nitrofurantoin	3	1.3	1.0	0.8						1.5		1.6	1.4	
Sulfonamides	5	2.2	1.6	1.4						1.4			1.2	

Figure 6-12 Maximum standard deviations in variability of precision allowable to maintain various probabilities that an isolate with a true zone diameter on the resistant edge of the indeterminate (or intermediate) zone would vary enough to appear susceptible, or the converse (after Gavan). Observed standard deviations from selected laboratories are shown. Column B is the Hartford Hospital laboratory.

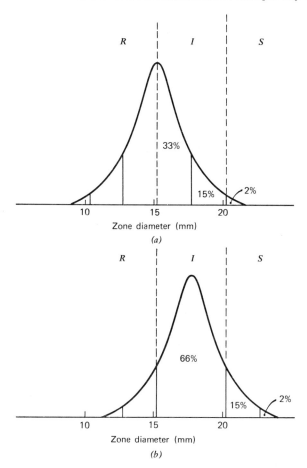

Figure 6-13   (a) Distribution of zone diameters observed with repeated antimicrobial suscepti-bility testing of an isolate by the method of Bauer et al. The mean or true value is assumed to coincide with the breakpoint between the resistant (R) and indeterminate (I) zones. If the standard deviation of the variability in precision of these analyses is one half the width of the indeterminate zone, 2% of the analyses will produce zone diameters in the susceptible (S) range. (b) Effect of error in the standardization of the procedure such that the mean is shifted by an amount equal to one half the width of the indeterminate zone. This might result from too light an inoculum, pH deviation, or other factors (see text). The variability in precision is the same as in a. This will cause 17% of the observations to fall in the susceptible range.

observed mean shows a deviation from the "true value" by the same amount the probability of an erroneous report is increased to 17% (Figure 6-13).

More advanced programs may make use of computers for analyzing this control data. In our laboratory Mueller-Hinton medium is tested prior to its use in the laboratory. The 60 values that are obtained from testing five inde-pendent cultures of the two control strains against six drugs are entered on a teletype. Acceptability is computed automatically. Instructions are im-mediately printed advising technologists of which drug results are to be withheld (Figure 6-14). If zones are unacceptable, large resistance is

```
E COLI
    AMP      17    19    18    17    17
    CEPH     23    23    22    23    23
    CHLORO   25    25    24    24    24
    POLY     18    18    19    19    19
    GENT     24    23    23    24    23
    KANA     24    22    23    24    22
    STREP    19    19    19    19    19
    TETRA    22    21    22    23    23

S. AUREUS
    CEPH     20    20    28    29    29
    CHLORO   23    22    22    21    21
    ERYTH    26    25    25    25    26
    METH     19    20    19    19    19
    PEN      29    30    29    29    29
    TETRA    24    25    24    23    24
```

		ACCURACY		PRECISION
	FDA MEAN	OBS MEAN	DIFFER	RANGE
E. COLI				
AMP	17.50	17.60	0.10	2
CEPH	20.50	22.80*	2.30	1
CHLORO	24.	24.40	0.40	1
POLY	13	18.40*	5.40	1
GENT	22.50	23.40	0.90	1
KANA	21	23	2	2
STREP	16	18.40	2.40	1
TETRA	21.50	22.20	0.70	2
S AUREUS				
CEPH	31	28.60	-2.40	1
CHLORO	22.50	21.80	- 0.70	2
ERYTH	26	25.40	-0.60	1
METH	19.50	19.20	-0.30	1
PEN	31.50	28.80	-2.70	2
TETRA	23.50	24	0.50	2

RESULTS WITH *, IF ANY ARE UNACCEPTABLE

```
DO NOT REPORT RESULTS WITH "X" MARK FOR 12/03/72

              SENS.      RES.
    CEPH       X
    POLY       X
```

Figure 6-14 Five values obtained from replicate tests of each control culture against antibiotics in use in the author's laboratory are entered in computer program by technologist. The system then prints a comparison of the observed mean, the FDA mean, and the range of precision variation. Unacceptable results are based on Gavan's data (see Figure 6-11) and are given an asterisk. After the page perforation is passed, the computer prints instructions to the technologist not to report results that may be erroneous. This is torn off and posted at the bench. See Figure AI-5, page 220, for a surveillance report of this observation.

154

Acceptable		19
Precision unacceptable		0
Accuracy unacceptable		17
Zone too small		
Cephalothin	2	
Chloramphenicol	10	
Colistin	2	
Gentamicin	2	
Zone too large		
Colistin	3	
Tetracycline	3	

Figure 6-15   Results of monitoring 36 batches of Mueller-Hinton medium with Seattle control cultures for precision and accuracy by Gavan's method.

reported but susceptibility is not. If zones are unacceptably small, the converse directions are given. Over a period of 4 months results with one or more drugs were withheld on *one half* of the batches of Mueller-Hinton medium that was prepared (Figure 6-15). This caused only occasional inquiries from clinicians who appeared more reassured by the use of controls than annoyed at the omission of results.

Other measures may be taken in *more complete* programs to control the quality of antimicrobial susceptibility testing data. Most microbiologists become accustomed to the antimicrobial susceptibility "profiles" displayed by various species (Figure 6-16). When unexpected results are obtained the susceptibility test and speciation of the isolate may be repeated. Many laboratories compile statistical reports of the susceptibility of common isolates to drugs being tested. These are quite useful to clinicians for selecting drugs prior to receiving results on individual specimens. A commercial program is available which calculates profiles for individual hospitals and compares the data with other institutions and national results. Unfortunately this data is collected from laboratories performing a wide variety of modifications of the method of Bauer et al. This has resulted in the reporting of improbabilities, such as *Hemophilus influenzae* resistant to ampicillin, and *Streptococcus pyogenes* resistant to penicillin.

A *more advanced* approach might make use of a computer program to establish acceptable profiles and automatically reject misfits. In our laboratory such a program maintains a rotating file of profiles for the most recent 50–100 isolates of common species. Patterns that occur less frequently than three times in the rotating file are rejected. Speciation and test results prove to be correct in 75% of the rejects and these are inserted in the computer file as verified results. The remaining 25% contain errors consisting of misspeciation, susceptibility testing errors, and mixed cultures. Of all drug results, 15–20% are rejected by this system. This represents the detection of errors in 4–5% of all reports. Reports are not withheld because of computer rejection. If a change results from repeat testing a supplementary report is sent to the chart with a note drawing attention to the correction. The system can provide substantial savings in unnecessary effort for speciation. For several years our computer file has shown over half of the *Escherichia coli* isolates susceptible to all drugs tested. Only infrequent isolates of *Citrobacter freundii* among other lactose fermenting species gives this profile. We believe this justifies reporting presumptive isolates of *Escherichia coli* that show susceptibility to all drugs tested without supplemental biochemical tests.

Petrali and his associates have published a similar approach in which zone diameter measurements are entered rather than S, I, or R as in our system (8). The program uses Bayes theorem to determine the probability of fit

ANTIBIOTIC SUSCEPTIBILITY PROFILE

PERCENT SUSCEPTIBILITY OF RECENTLY ISOLATED CULTURES
HARTFORD HOSPITAL 08/24/72

SPECIES	AMP	CEP	ERY	GEN	KAN	LIN	OXA	PEN	POL	STR	TET	TOTAL
CITROBACTER	8	22		98	98				100	58	88	(50)
ENTEROBACTER	8	7		100	80				92	76	75	(100)
E. COLI	87	84		100	94				99	79	79	(100)
HERELLEA	4	0		94	95				94	70	70	(92)
KLEBSIELLA	0	94		100	96				100	96	94	(100)
MIMA	56	19		87	81				56	81	50	(16)
PROT. MIRAB	94	98		100	96				1	85	2	(100)
PROT. MORG	2	0		100	98				2	90	78	(50)
PROT. RETT	12	8		96	96				4	28	0	(25)
PROT. VULG.	5	2		100	100				0	97	56	(37)
PROVIDENCIA	25	4		91	87				4	16	8	(24)
PSEUDOMONAS	2	2		97	3				99	2	4	(100)
SERRATIA	0	0		100	36				13	16	0	(100)
ENTEROCOCCUS	100	5	61			3	0	13			13	(100)
STAPH. AUREUS		100	97			100	99	23			98	(100)
STAPH. EPIDERM.		99	91			98	95	30			61	(100)

Figure 6-16 Computer printout of antibiotic susceptibility profiles. This is distributed to the medical staff for guidance in therapy. It is also a component of a system for automatic rejection by the computer of isolates that do not fit the expected pattern.

with the data base. They found errors in 15% of the reports with this system. Other workers are experimenting with related computer applications for quality control and bacterial speciation.

A survey conducted by the Connecticut State Department of Health revealed lack of agreement in testing unknown cultures in 50 laboratories in 1968 (Figure 17). A recent survey has shown marked improvement.

DILUTION METHODS OF ANTIMICROBIAL SUSCEPTIBILITY TESTING (BASIC)

Stock cultures should be maintained to assure reproducibility of performance as a *basic* control measure in laboratories performing this test. An enterococcus strain is used in our laboratory each time dilution suscepti-

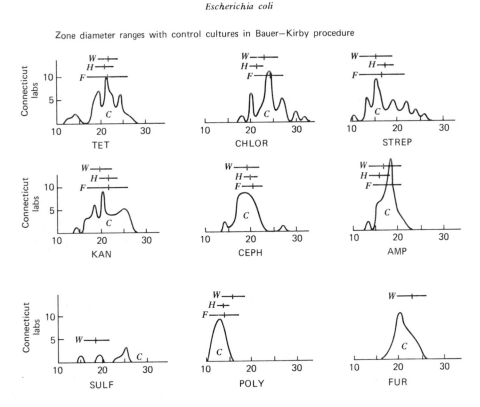

Escherichia coli

Zone diameter ranges with control cultures in Bauer–Kirby procedure

Figure 6-17   Results of testing control cultures for disk susceptibility in two hospital laboratories, a study conducted by the FDA in 14 selected hospital laboratories and a survey of 50 laboratories in Connecticut conducted by the Connecticut State Department of Health. Note the wide range of results in the state survey indicating the need for improved control of the procedure. *W* = University of Washington control data. *H* = Hartford Hospital Control data. *F* = FDA study of 14 labs. *C* = Connecticut Survey of 50 labs.

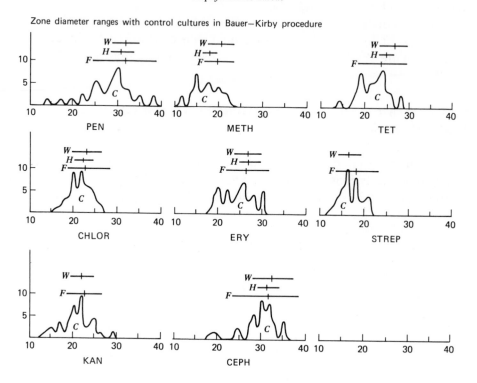

Figure 6-17 (cont.)

bility tests are conducted using penicillin. If results deviate by more than one tube from the expected minimum inhibitory concentration the test is repeated.

OVERALL SURVEILLANCE OF SUSCEPTIBILITY TEST CONTROL ACTIVITIES (BASIC)

Surveillance must include periodic checks to assure that all of the control measures that have been established are being conducted as scheduled. This provides assurance that control cultures are used regularly, reporting is interrupted if controls are unacceptable, investigation of unacceptable control results is documented, unacceptable profiles are repeated, and so forth. Any omission of these regular control procedures or any deficiencies found are documented and reported to the director in the periodic surveillance report.

REAGENTS (BASIC, MORE COMPLETE)

Control of the duration and storage conditions of reagents through an inventory as a portion of a *basic* control program is discussed on page 129. Testing may be conducted when freshly prepared reagents are placed in use or intermittently during the accepted duration of their use. This problem is similar to that encountered with media and is dealt with differently in large and small laboratories. In a *basic* control program reagents may be tested as they are received or prepared, or only intermittently if they are unstable, for example, an oxidase test; or if the tests are performed too infrequently to assure valid interpretation.

Infrequently used biologicals required for serological procedures should be evaluated in a *more complete* program by performing tests at least once a month, even if no clinical request for performance has been received. This consumes control materials and reagents that would otherwise become outdated and require replacement, and simultaneously maintains proficiency of personnel.

Staining reagents should be tested frequently in a *basic* control program, not so much as a test of the stain as for a test of procedure and interpretation. Monitoring the Gram stain by known Gram positive and Gram negative organisms is a waste of time if sight is lost of the pitfalls. Overdecolorization of old cultures and underdecolorization of thick smears are a more significant source of misinterpretation than defective reagents. Known positive smears of acid-fast bacilli should be included with each batch of smears for Ziehl-Neilsen or Rhodamine-auramine staining. These should be made from positive clinical specimens, not cultures. The latter contain too many organisms to represent a realistic control. Furthermore, organisms may fall off and transfer to other slides, resulting in false positives. Never stain smears of cultures and body fluids at the same time for the same reason.

Procedure book descriptions of all analytical procedures must include use of control materials. In general it must be established in any *basic* control program that any chemical, immunologic, or staining reaction be controlled by known positive and negative materials at established frequencies, if not every time they are used. When controls deviate from the expected value by more than one two fold dilution, results should be reported with the comment "Control data erratic—test being repeated." A supplementary report is rendered when control results become acceptable. Two positive coded control sera of slightly different activity unknown to the worker may be used to reduce bias. Workers must take their results to the supervisor or quality control specialist to decode the unknown control and determine the acceptability of the results (Figures 6-18, 6-19, 6-20 and 6-21).

Antisera present the dual problem of evaluating reactivity and specificity. A conjugate used for identifying *Neisseria gonorrhoeae* by immuno-

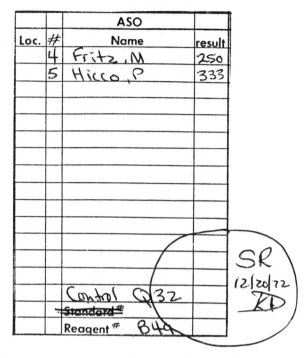

Figure 6-18 Technician omitted recording of control results in performance of antistreptolysin titer. Supervisor notes error and indicates that occurrence has been recorded in the surveillance report (SR). (See graphic display of control data in Figure 6-19 and surveillance report of incident in Figure AI-8).

fluorescence may be evaluated by testing one homologous and one heterologous species. To do the same with antisera used for grouping *Salmonella sp.* requires at least 25 separate combinations. Instead in a *basic* program stock cultures of each group may be tested with the homologous antiserum only. This may be done periodically or when new reagents are placed in use. The latter approach does not protect against contamination, accidental mixing, or dilution that could occur sometime during the laboratory life of the material. The thorough evaluation of serological reagents requires testing antigens with homologous and heterologous antisera (and the converse) in twofold dilution to establish specificity and reactivity. This is not practical even for advanced quality control programs in clinical laboratories to perform. Instead, manufacturers must be required to assure that reagents comply with CDC specifications, which establish proper specificity and reactivity. A complete discussion of this problem appears on page 65 in Chapter 3. Control measures used in clinical laboratories must of necessity be only superficially confirmatory.

The surveillance schedule must establish a monitoring system to assure that reagents were tested according to an established schedule and that any defects were recorded and corrected. For example, someone must check to

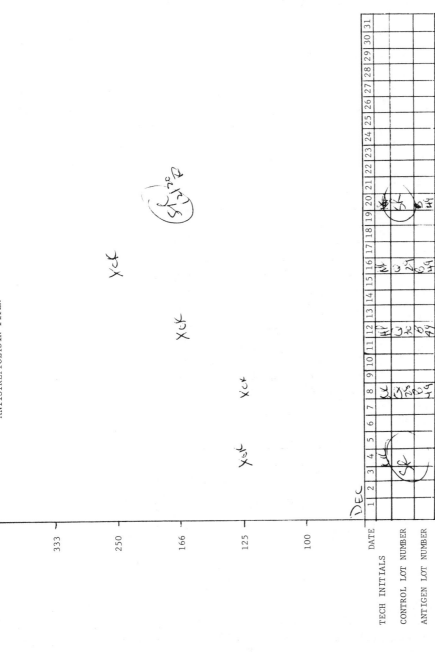

Figure 6-19 Technician did not record the control and antigen lot numbers although control results were recorded on 12/4/72. On 12/20/72 she omitted the control number and failed to record the results. The control number was entered on the day sheet (see Figure 6-18) but she apparently forgot to test it. These errors are documented in the surveillance report (see Figure AI-8). Coded controls give different results which the technician must clear with the supervisor before reporting. OK indicates that the supervisor approved the results.

161

see that each batch of smears for acid-fast bacilli contains a positive control smear. It might be a good idea to look at the control smear. We have had the experience of observing reports of positive results on control smears in which we could find no organisms. The truth of the matter as expressed by one technician could weaken the most resolute supervisor—"well if you look really hard you may be able to find a bug but I knew it was supposed to be positive, so I called it."

It is necessary to check that infrequently performed serologic tests are being conducted once a month if this is a part of the program. We have had repeated difficulty with personnel who perform serologic tests without controls, do not record control results, and fail to repeat tests when controls are unacceptable. The system must detect these irregularities and summarize them in a periodic *surveillance report*.

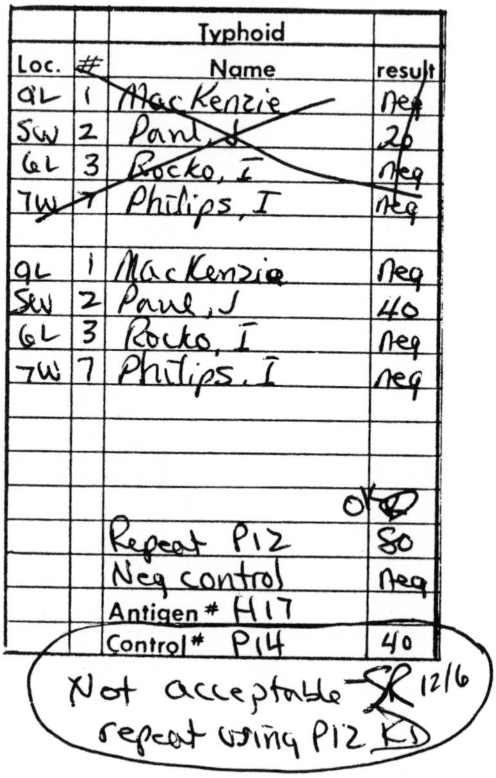

Figure 6-20 Portion of the daysheet used for recording results on immunologic tests, in this case Typ[h]oid O. Observed titer of 40 on control P14 was unacceptable (mean titer of P14 was 160, see Figu[re] 6-21). The supervisor indicated that tests should be repeated using another control, P12. The corre[ct] result was obtained. Note the correction in result on patient serum. The supervisor approved th[e] reporting of results when the correct control value was obtained. Results were reported on the sam[e] day (see Figure 6-21 for a graphic display of this data). Figure AI-9, p. 224, represents a report of th[is] incident in the monthly surveillance report.

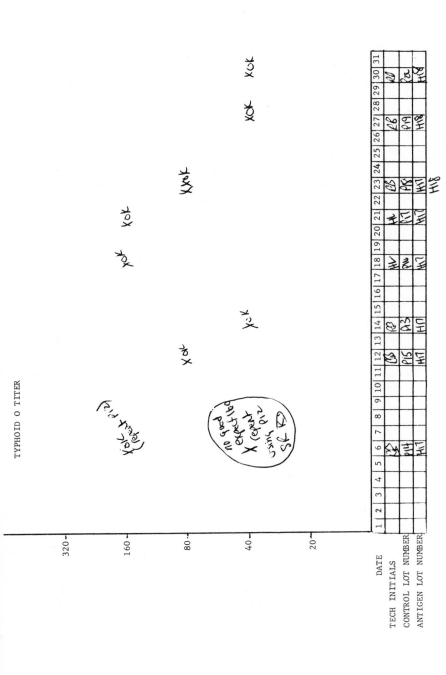

Figure 6-21 Graphic display of control results for Typhoid O titer. Technician enters the result on the day sheet (Figure 6-20) with numbers identifying the control and reagents used. The technician does not know the expected control result. This must be approved by the supervisor before reporting. An erroneous control result was obtained on 12/6/72. The supervisor instructed the technologist to use another control P12, because P14 had yielded incorrect results. Note that correct results were obtained with P12. The incident is documented in the monthly surveillance report (see Figure AI-9, p. 224). Note the testing of a new reagent on 12/23 with the reagent previously in use. This assures that expected control results will be obtained before the old reagent is exhausted.

163

MEDIA (BASIC; MORE ADVANCED; MORE COMPLETE)

Surveillance of the quality of media looms as an apparently insurmountable task to those who have not entered into it in a gradual and systematic fashion. The need to establish a *basic* program is a high priority item when starting quality control activities in microbiology. This is affirmed by the frequency with which defective media are observed in clinical laboratories. Although commercial suppliers are applying controls to their products we, and other workers who have studied the problem, have found a higher incidence of defects in commercial media than in media produced in our own laboratories. In some cases media may be acceptable when they leave the manufacturer but deteriorate in shipping and storage. It is essential that controls be applied to commercially prepared as well as "home made" media.

There are features of basic media control that are often overlooked in the haste to establish testing with stock cultures. In the discussion of the inventory earlier in this chapter, the need to define and monitor the limits of time and conditions of storage for dehydrated and prepared media was stressed (see p. 132). Weighing errors are easily made, especially if small amounts are being prepared. Improper or insufficient mixing may result in heterogeneous suspensions which, when distributed into tubes, yield media of inconsistent composition. Some highly inhibitory media, such as SS, do not require autoclaving and are damaged by it. Desoxycholate must be added to XLD medium *after* autoclaving. It is well known that disaccharides may hydrolyze when autoclaved. Solutions and media containing these carbohydrates should be filtered. Hospital engineering and maintenance personnel assume that autoclaves are designed to kill bacteria and that a little higher temperature will assure even better performance. The minimal bacterial contamination of fresh media requires only a brief exposure. Most media are brought to too high a temperature for too long. Spore suspensions should not be used to monitor a media autoclave because optimal con-

	Thermocouple Measurements Inside Vessel			Temperature $\geq 121°C$ at Exhaust Valve
	$< 121°C$ Heating	$\geq 121°C$ Sterilization	$< 121°C$ Cooling	
Tubes	2	12	20	34
Flask (1000 ml)	12	12	30	54
Flask (2000 ml)	20	12	40	72

Figure 6-22 Duration of exposure to heat increases with the volume of fluid. To assure but limit exposure of the media to 12 minutes at 121°C, the total time at this temperature, measured at the exhaust valve, requires experimental thermocouple measurements made in the vessel inside the autoclave. Alternatively, published guidelines may be used.

MEDIA CONTROL SHEET

Med Decarboxylase, lysine   pH 5.4 ± 0.2

Date	Bottle Code	Vol	Units pH	pH	T >121 C°	T >100 C°	E. coli K O A	Enterobacter K O A	Pseudomonas K O A
12/15	10	4	10	6.0	9	30	X (SR)	(A)	(O) X
12/16	11	7	25	6.0	10	35	X	X	X
12/21	10	7	25	5.8	22 SR 12/21	45	X	X	X
12/28	11	7	100 (12/28)	5.6					
12/28	11	7	100	6.0	9	25	X	X	X

Figure 6-23 Media control sheet used to record observations from surveillance of media preparation and function. Notice the sequential use of coded bottles of dehydrated material. Coding bottles assists in detecting sources of variability that might result from a change in a batch of dehydrated media. The volume determines the maximum exposure time for temperatures of 121 and 100°C. (See Surveillance Schedule, VIII, A, Autoclave cycles p. 192.) Reactions with control cultures are: K = alkaline; O = no change; A = acid. A number of errors were noted and recorded in the surveillance report (SR). On 12/15 the batch failed to give the expected alkaline reaction with *Escherichia coli*. On 12/21 excessive autoclaving occurred. On 12/28 the pH was too low and the batch was not noted on the chart from the time temperature recorder on the autoclave. See Figure AI-10, page 225, for surveillance report on these incidents.

ditions for media preparation will probably not sterilize it. Figure 6-22 illustrates the striking differences in time required to heat, sterilize, and cool off solutions in containers of varying size. Separate standards must be established to bring the medium to a temperature not exceeding 121°C for a maximum of 12 minutes. Regular cleaning of autoclaves is necessary to prevent accumulation of dirt which will delay the exhaust cycle. Properly calibrated time temperature recorders should be used to verify the correct autoclaving of each batch of media. Someone should check these regularly to assure that proper exposure was given for the volume of media processed. The temperature of media to which blood is added for preparing chocolate agar must be controlled. A thermometer that is stored in 70% alcohol may be used to assure the addition of blood at about 45°C. A water bath kept at this temperature may also be of assistance.

The pH of all media should be tested after it has been poured into a small container and brought to room temperature (Figure 6-23). The pH changes during autoclaving and as temperature changes. Calibration of pH meters for higher temperatures is technically undesirable. Any pH meter and electrode may be used. Solid media may be removed from tubes or plates with a spatula and ground into a slurry in a mortar or beaker so that measurements can be taken with conventional immersion electrodes. Alternatively, a surface electrode may be used, but these are expensive and easily damaged. Media room personnel can be taught to use pH meters and, by trial and error, to compute the amount of acid or base needed to correct a subsequent batch. Batches that exceed optimum pH by more than ± 0.2 pH units are discarded in our laboratory. Correction is made by adding $0.1N$ HCl and NaOH. Only a few milliters are required, hence this does not significantly dilute other components of the medium. Indicator solutions and paper test strips are not suitable for testing the pH of media.

Uneven thickness of agar plates occurs if slanted or irregular surfaces are used. Large marble slabs are a good cure for warped table tops. A uniform thickness is important with Mueller-Hinton medium for susceptibility testing (4–6 mm) and blood agar plates (3 mm). The length of a slant should equal the length of the butt, and no tube should be filled more than two-thirds.

Ten percent of all batches of noninhibitory media, such as blood agar and chocolate agar, should be incubated for evidence of contamination prior to releasing the media for use. This may be extended to other media if contamination problems are encountered. These media should be discarded because of the drying effects of incubation. Some media require drying with lids "cracked open" prior to refrigeration, especially if they are bagged. Otherwise condensation occurs causing the growth to spread on the plates. Incubation of such plates is a less desirable way of controlling the condensation problem.

Other observations may be made including the appearance of precipitates, bubbles, and unexpected colors from visual inspection of media. Tubes that have been inoculated with a sterile loop or wire should be used for comparison with inoculated tubes by all personnel in daily work. Many an "alkaline" TSI has been called "alkaline over acid" when comparison with an uninoculated tube could have revealed the change as one of only increasing alkalinity in the slant. Tubes with tight closures, including screw caps, should not be used if oxidation is an important element of the reaction to take place in the medium.

Testing of media with stock cultures may follow the *basic* controls reviewed in previous paragraphs. Priorities may be assigned according to the clinical significance of errors that might result from using a deficient medium combined with the observed frequency of error experienced in established surveillance programs (See figures 6-24, 6-25 and 6-27). Failure to isolate *Neisseria gonorrhoeae* because of defective chocolate agar is more serious than misspeciation of *Candida* because of defective corn meal agar. Media may be divided into three categories on this basis. Figure 6-26 lists cultures that may be employed for the surveillance of media. Relative priorities are provided. Fourteen cultures are required for monitoring first priority media in a *basic* quality control program. An additional six are required for second priority media in a *more complete* program. A total of 28 are required for a *more advanced* program which monitors all media.

STOCK CULTURES (BASIC)

Stock cultures may be obtained from the American Type Culture Collection; other sources include proficiency testing programs, regional reference laboratories, and laboratory supply houses (Figure 6-28). Cultures may be shipped on slants, in lyophile, or on paper disks or strips. Lyophilized cultures in bottles that are reconstituted by injecting water or broth may be handled without a hood, but a cotton pledget should be held at the junction of the cap and the needle to prevent production of aerosol when the needle is withdrawn. Ampules that must be broken prior to the reconstitution of cultures must only be opened in a properly functioning safety hood containing an ultrafilter or an air incinerator. Cultures should be grown in suitable nutrient broth and later streaked on solid media to assure viability and purity. Figure 6-29 tabulates many methods that are successful for maintaining cultures in the laboratory. Liquid nitrogen is less expensive than lyophilization, but labor and amortization of equipment results in a cost of 1 or 2 dollars per container when processed by either of these techniques. They are practical only if upward of a hundred stock strains are maintained for quality control, development and educational purposes.

Media	Source	Number of Batches	Frequency of Times	Percentage	Nature of Problem
Columbia selective agar	M, C	145	39	27	Poor or no growth with wild staphylococcus; failure to inhibit *Pseudomonas*.
OF-maltose	M	14	3	2	*P. maltophilia* negative, pH off, contamination.
Selenite broth	M, C	74	8	11	No growth of *Salmonella*, no inhibition of *E. coli*, contaminated with Gram negative rods 6 times.
KCN	M	51	5	10	Growth of *Shigella* control, *Salmonella* positive three times.
Chocolate agar	M, C	134	13	9.7	Poor growth of *N. gonorrhoeae*, contamination.
OF-dextrose	M	71	6	8	No agar in medium, contaminated, too light, pH off, no oxidation by *P. aeruginosa*
Thayer-Martin	M, C	63	3	5	No Supplement B added, poor growth of *N. gonorrhoeae* twice.
Eosin-methylene blue	C	160	8	5	Poor lactose reactions, color differences.
Sugars	M	201	7	4	Too red, too light, contaminated batch, too much indicator, media solidified.
Lysine iron agar	C	88	3	3	Agar not dissolved, reactions hard to read, no deaminase reaction.
Sabouraud's	C	97	3	3	Poor *Candida* growth, *E. coli* not inhibited three times.
Salmonella-Shigella	C	95	3	3	Media too soft, poor growth *Salmonella* twice.
Horse blood selective	M	67	2	3	*H. influenzae* grew poorly, plates too dark.
Citrate	C	108	2	2	Alkaline reaction weak, poor growth *Klebsiella*.
DNase agar	M	115	2	2	Media too dark, hard to read positives.

Media					
Ornithine broth	C	50	1	2	Enterobacter control not very purple.
Phenyl ethyl alcohol	M, C	99	2	2	No inhibition of *E. coli*, media too old.
Thioglycollate	M	130	2	2	Not enough agar in tubes.
Blood agar slant	M	120	2	1.7	Whole batch contaminated twice.
Brain heart infusion	M	68	1	1.5	*H. influenzae* failed to grow.
Hektoen agar	C	68	1	>1	No growth of *Shigella*.
MacConkey	C	136	1	>1	All colonies have fringy edges.
Mold inhibitory	M	150	1	>1	Media too liquid.
Motility indol-ornithine	M	108	1	>1	Agar not distributed evenly.
Sheep blood agar	C	335	2	<1	Deep contaminating colonies, media frozen (average contamination rate about 1%).
X-L-D	C	76	1	<1	*Salmonella* too yellow.
Blood culture bottles	M	—	2		Agar poorly distributed (0.15% agar).
Mueller-Hinton agar	C	—	5		pH 6.2, excessive contamination.
Triple sugar iron	C	325	0	0	

M—prepared in University of Minnesota Laboratory. C—prepared in commercial laboratory.

Figure 6-24 Media deficiency problems encountered at the University of Minnesota Hospital laboratory. (Courtesy of John M. Matsen, Donna J. Blazevic, and Marilyn H. Koepcke, University of Minnesota.) Note the high frequency of problems with Columbia selective agar, OF-maltose, and Selenite broth and the low frequency of problems with TSI, XLD, and MacConkey. Monitoring should be concentrated on media that give the most trouble and omitted when deficiencies are rarely if ever observed.

We have found that maintaining fastidious organisms, such as *Hemophilus influenzae, D. pneumoniae,* and *Neisseria gonorrhoeae*, is practical on chocolate agar plates kept in a capneic incubator and transferred every 4 days. Other cultures are grown on nutrient agar slants, transferred once a week, and kept at room temperature. Anaerobes are kept at room temperature in chopped meat broth and are subcultured every 2–3 months.

IMPLEMENTING SURVEILLANCE WITH STOCK CULTURES (BASIC)

In a large laboratory, such as ours, the duty of monitoring each batch of medium with stock cultures may be distributed among all personnel or performed by one person whose primary responsibility is quality control. We tried both approaches and found the second more satisfactory because of the dispersion of effort involved and the sense of participation in quality control that it gives to all workers. In a large laboratory it is not difficult to prepare batches of media that will be consumed well within the expiration date. In smaller laboratories the burden of testing may fall on one person. The question arises also whether the media should be tested when they are made or received, when they are used, or both. If they are tested when made or received, there is no assurance that they will function properly weeks or months later. If media are tested when they are used, it is too late to find out that they do not work! Testing them both times is burdensome. In small laboratories performing limited bacteriology, as much media might be used for quality control as for testing specimens. There is evidence that most of the defects that occur in media result from improper preparation and that storage in airtight bags at controlled temperatures will preserve the function unchanged for weeks or months. Therefore, first priority should be given to testing media when they are made or received. Another consideration may be the lack of familiarity with interpretation if media are infrequently used.

Autoclave time and temperature		
Maximum exceeded	345	13%
Minimum not achieved	13	<1%
Control information not recorded	89	3%
In use beyond expiration date	58	2%
Control culture results unacceptable	28	1%
pH of media $> \pm 0.2$	27	1%
Appearance of media unacceptable	17	<1%
Contamination of media	16	<1%
Improper storage	11	<1%

Figure 6-25   Errors or deficiencies detected in a surveillance of the quality of 2700 batches of media prepared in the author's laboratory between 6/2/71 and 1/14/73.

Media

First priority	Second priority
Blood agar	MacConkey
Chocolate agar	PEA
Thayer-Martin	XLD
Martin Lester	Urea
TSI	Decarboxylase
	Thioglycollate

Third priority

GN broth	Rice plate
MRVP broth	DN'ase
ONPG	SIM
PSE	Citrate
Blood broth	Transport
Soy	TSN
6.5% NaCl	Carbohydrates
Gelatin	Indole-nitrate

Stocks

First priority	Second priority
S. aureus (susceptibility test control)	S. flexneri
E. coli (susceptibility test control)	K. pneumoniae
Group A Streptococcus	P. mirabilis
S. viridans	C. novyii
H. influenzae	S. viridans
N. meningitidis	Enterococcus
N. gonorrhoeae	
S. aureus	Third priority
E. coli	
C. albicans	Candida sp. (not albicans)
D. pneumoniae	Serratia
S. typhimurium	S. epidermidis
P. rettgeri	C. perfringens
Ps. aeruginosa	P. morganii
	P. maltophilia
	Arizona
	Herellea

Figure 6-26 First priority media represent those that are sometimes deficient and are essential to primary isolation and differentiation of important pathogens. Second priority includes those less likely to be deficient and of less importance in primary isolation and differentiation. Third priority are media that infrequently are deficient and are not crucial to primary isolation and differentiation. First priority media require 14 stock cultures for monitoring. The complete list requires 28 cultures. See the surveillance schedule in Appendix I for a more complete list of media and stock cultures.)

If media are used only once or twice a month, it would be prudent to require that controls be run with them.

Solid media are streaked with inoculum taken directly from stock cultures by a loop or straight wire using a sector method that produces isolated colonies. We have attempted to dilute stock cultures to provide a lighter inoculum, but this has introduced additional time-consuming steps of doubtful value. The criticism is well taken that the ability of a massive ino-

Media	Batches	Contaminated	Control Culture Results Unacceptable	Unacceptable Appearance	pH > ±0.2	Total Deficient	Percentage
Martin-Lester	33	0	15	0	0	15	45
Blood broth	48	1	0	Hemolyzed 14	0	15	31
Mycobiotic	36	0	3	0	3	6	17
Malonate	36	0	0	0	3	3	8
Salt broth	50	0	0	0	3	3	6
Transport	35	0	0	0	2	2	6
Chocolate	164	6	2	0	0	8	5
Biplates	135	5	2	0	0	7	5
Thio	202	0	0	0	9	9	4
Decarboxylase lysine	38	0	1	0	0	1	3
BAP	180	4	1	0	0	5	3
Citrate	58	0	0	0	2	2	3
Mueller-Hinton	131	0	[a]	0	4	4[a]	3[a]
VCN	94	0	0	1	1	2	2
MacConkey	117	0	2	0	0	2	2
OF	59	0	1	0	0	1	2
Sab	46	0	[b]	0	1	1	2
Todd-Hewitt	41	0	1	0	1	1	2
TSB	90	0	1	0	0	1	1

Urea	57	0	0	0	0	0	0
CTA	34	0	0	0	0	0	0
Decarboxylase base	50	0	0	0	0	0	0
Decarboxylase ornithine	43	0	0	0	0	0	0
DN²ase	34	0	0	0	0	0	0
GN broth	42	0	0	0	0	0	0
Indole nitrate	50	0	0	0	0	0	0
MRVP	38	0	0	0	0	0	0
PAD	9	0	0	0	0	0	0
PEA	65	0	0	0	0	0	0
PSE	51	0	0	0	0	0	0
Pseudosel	28	0	0	0	0	0	0
Rice	19	0	b	0	0	0	0
Rodac	31	0	0	0	0	0	0
SIM	48	0	0	0	0	0	0
TSA	92	0	0	0	0	0	0
TSI	58	0	0	0	0	0	0
TSN	24	0	0	0	0	0	0
XLD	58	0	0	0	0	0	0
Total	2424	16	28	16	27	87	3.6

[a] Monitored separately for conformance to disk susceptibility test criteria.
[b] Control cultures not tested.

Figure 6-27 Deficiencies observed in a surveillance of various types of media prepared in the author's laboratory between 6/2/71 and 1/14/7

A Proficiency testing programs
   (1) State and federal
   (2) CAP
B Check sample program ASCP
C Regional reference laboratories
D American Type Culture Collection
   12301 Parklawn Drive
   Rockville, Maryland 20852
E Commercial Laboratory Supply Houses
   (1) Difco Laboratories
      920 Henry Street
      Detroit, Michigan 48201
   (2) Hyland Laboratories
      3300 Hyland Avenue
      Costa Mesa, California 92926
   (3) Roche Diagnostics
      Nutley, New Jersey 07110

Figure 6-28   Sources of stock cultures.

culum of laboratory adapted strains to grow is not a test of whether a medium can isolate small numbers of pathogens from clinical material. On the other hand, defective media that assuredly would not support the growth of fastidious clinical isolates will be detected by this technique.

The surveillance system must include systematic checks on the media monitoring program. These are listed in the surveillance schedule in the appendix. It is essential to assure that established standards for media preparation are maintained and that irregularities are documented and corrected. Periodic checks must be made to assure that control cultures *are*

A CTA or carbohydrate free nutrient agar, 4–8°C or −5°C (general purpose: transfer every 2–4 weeks)
B. Skim milk, −20°C (transfer every 2–4 weeks)
   Neisseria sp.
C Blood agar slant, 4–8°C (transfer every 2 weeks)
   D. pneumoniae
   Streptococci
D Chocolate agar, 20 or −20°C (not 4–8°C)
   Hemophilus sp.⎫
   Neisseria sp.⎬ transfer once a week
E Chopped meat, 4–8°C or 20°C (transfer every 2–3 months)
   Enteric bacteria
   Micrococci
   Corynebacteria
   Bacteroides⎫
   Clostridia⎬ under oil
F Lyophilization
G Liquid nitrogen

Figure 6-29   Methods of maintaining stock cultures.

used and that media deficiencies *are* recorded and corrected. The importance of establishing this "surveillance over surveillance" cannot be overemphasized. Without it busy personnel may gradually discontinue media control measures and the program will require complete reconstruction by the time it is discovered.

BLIND UNKNOWNS (MORE COMPLETE AND MORE ADVANCED)

The preparation and processing of blind unknown specimens in microbiology is a challenging quality control measure suitable for *more complete* and *more advanced* quality control programs. It provides simultaneous testing of materials, validity of procedures, interpretative standards, and performance of personnel. Unfortunately it is difficult to apply in laboratories where less than two or three full-time workers are engaged in microbiology. In such instances it would be possible for several small laboratories in a related geographic area to prepare and submit specimens to each other. The different types of requisition slips and containers involved, as well as the elaborate logistics, has prevented such programs from being established.

In most hospitals it is possible to prepare requisition slips with pseudonyms. A complete explanation of the purpose of conducting such studies should be provided for administration and medical staff. Initial reactions in many hospitals have been to disapprove such a procedure either because of fear of legal entanglement or confusion on the part of physicians and nurses who might receive reports on nonexistent patients. Laboratory workers in numerous hospitals have surmounted this obstacle and have begun submitting specimens. It is not infrequent for reports to be returned to patient care units. We know of no instance in which this has resulted in any legal action, significantly confused physicians and nurses, or compromised patient care. When reports have escaped from our laboratory a simple explanation to a nurse or a physician has always resulted in a favorable reaction reflecting their recognition of the importance of conducting quality control in the laboratory. A "more complete" program may begin with bacteriologic specimens.

Blood and various body fluids including cavity, urine, and spinal fluids that are sterile may be used after the inoculation of highly diluted broth cultures of organisms to be submitted. Plain broth may be used to mimic urine specimens. We have found that workers rarely detect the difference in odor. Saline suspensions may be used for spinal fluid. These may be made more realistic by adding a few dabs of buffy coat. It is not necessary to emulsify feces with an inoculum of a test organism. Simply coating the exterior of a small amount of a feces specimen with a diluted culture usually provides a realistic culture. Wound cultures are more difficult to simulate and require the use of buffy coat material. Very often Gram stains of artificial wound exudates do not correlate with cultures and this causes undesired confusion in interpretation and reporting.

A number of points should be considered in evaluating the analysis of such specimens. A common problem in many laboratories is excessive delay, especially in the preliminary reporting of results on unusual isolates. We have frequently observed several days of delay prior to preliminary reporting, as well as excessive delay prior to delivering a final report. Application of minimum or standard criteria established in the procedure manual for individual species can be confirmed. One can determine whether these procedures were conducted efficiently and in the proper order. By maintaining some casual surveillance of the worker during the processing of blind specimens we have often observed test results that were incorrectly interpreted. This observation would have been missed if the evaluation were based only on an examination of the final report.

Although the supervisor may not prepare, submit, and observe the processing of a blind unknown, the results may be organized for ease in conducting a review with the worker involved (see Figures 6-30 and AI-4). It is important to provide praise and reassurance where good quality work is observed as well as criticism and correction where deficiencies are found. It is helpful if the names of workers who have demonstrated deficiencies in the handling of blind unknowns are not included in the *monthly surveillance report* to the director. The surveillance report should establish that blind unknowns were submitted according to schedule or why this was not accomplished, whether discrepancies occurred, and if so, whether they were resolved with the worker. In small laboratories anonymity is difficult to preserve. This adds to the difficulty of conducting such studies in small laboratories. Even in large laboratories personnel may be sensitive about being subjected to such evaluations. Although this was an initial response in the author's laboratory, a curious reaction ensued. Workers became accustomed to an increase in the appearance of unusual isolates. Although they knew that some of these might be blind unknowns it decreased the ratio between commonplace isolates and those providing more of a challenge. When blind unknowns were not being submitted because of problems that interfered with their preparation and processing personnel expressed disappointment! For examples of blind unknowns which were correctly identified see figure 6-31.

Many interesting pitfalls may be observed in examining the results of blind unknowns. Inadequate criteria for the separation of *Serratia* from delayed or nonlactose fermenting variants of other members of the *Klebsiella, Enterobacter* group became apparent from one of the early blinds submitted in our laboratory. This resulted in replacement of gelatin liquification by tests for arabinose fermentation and DNase production. Misinterpretation of decolorized Gram positive rods as Gram negative rods was commonly observed. A series of blind unknowns helped make personnel aware of a common error, assuming that Gram positive rods found in anaerobic broth were *Bacillus sp.* when *Bacillus sp.* were observed on plates. This resulted in a failure to identify *Clostridium sp.* in thioglycollate broths from several specimens (Figure 6-32). The glib treatment of nonhemolytic nonmotile *Bacillus sp.* was abruptly terminated by the submission of a *Bacillus anthracis* culture that was promptly reported as a *Bacillus sp.*! Familiarity of personnel with isolating and identifying significant but infrequent isolates such as *Brucella sp., Pseudomonas cepaciae, Vibrio parahemolyticus, Yersinia enterocolitica,* and *Listeria monocytogenes* is periodically reassurred through this means.

Submission of consistently obscure and difficult isolates as blind unknowns will discourage workers. In the initial phases of such a program it would be preferable to submit a substantial number of commonplace isolates. A description of techniques for maintaining stock cultures that may be used for preparing blind unknowns is found in the discussion of media monitoring (see p. 170). The collection of obscure and unusual isolates would represent a lower order of priority than the collection of the basic cultures required for monitoring media and initiating a blind unknown program.

In a *"more advanced"* program not only very unusual species but also blind unknowns in other areas of microbiology may be submitted. We have an arrangement with a nearby sanitarium to submit to us periodic sputum specimens known to demonstrate acid-fast bacilli. Nail and skin scrapings can be collected from patients with established fungal infections. This material may be preserved in tightly stoppered containers and submitted as blind unknowns.

Serum may be submitted for blind unknown serological tests. If these tests are always received in the form of clotted blood samples, the submission of sera may bias the worker. In many laboratories, including our own, serum is removed from clots in other laboratory divisions for the performance of other tests and the serum is transferred to microbiology. If personnel realize that blind unknowns are always received in this fashion, this will also provide some bias. Results of blind unknowns submitted in the author's serology subdivision have shown perfect agreement with expected results, suggesting some undetected element of bias.

During the past 5 years more than 2000 blind unknown urinary sediments have been submitted to our personnel. This has been achieved by splitting specimens that demonstrate abnormal chemical screening test results or microscopic findings and resubmitting them with a pseudonym. The results are subsequently correlated by a supervisor and discrepancies are reviewed with the technologists involved. This has provided a unique element of discipline in the performance of a test that is easily performed in a slipshod fashion. We have observed astonishing discrepancies, including the failure to find

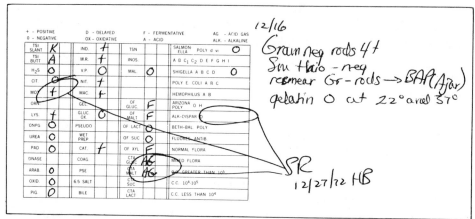

Figure 6-30 Report and laboratory file copies of blind unknowns are copied with a stock culture card for ease of comparing observations. Results that disagree with stock culture cards are repeated by the supervisor to assure that the culture gives expected reactions and for the instruction of the technologist who made errors in processing. See the surveillance report in Appendix I (Figure AI-4, p. 219).

178

1	*Proteus sp.*	Blood
2	*S. aureus*	Urine
3	Nonhemolytic streptococcus	Chest fluid
4	*Citrobacter*	Wound
5	*M. polymorpha*	Urine
6	*L. monocytogenes*	Blood
7	*H. aphrophilus*	Blood
8	*Salmonella* group A	Feces
9	*Providence (P. inconstans)*	Urine
10	"Bethesda-Ballerup" *Citrobacter*	Feces
11	*Moraxella var.* nonliquefaciens	Eye
12	*A. fecalis*	Blood
13	*Salmonella* group C_2	Feces
14	*E. aerogenes*	Blood
15	Smear for AFB	Smear
16	*K. pneumoniae*	Eye
17	*Salmonella* group C_2	Feces
18	*Ps. stutzeri*	Wound
19	*E. tarda*	Fluid
20	*B. anthracis*	Wound
21	*B. suis*	Blood
22	*Lophomonas sp.*	Fluid
23	*S. typhi*	Gall bladder bile
24	*E. tarda*	Urine
25	*Providencia*	Fluid
26	Enteropathogenic *E. coli*	Feces
27	Group A beta hemolytic streptococcus	Throat
28	*K. pneumoniae*	Urine
29	*Aeromonas sp.*	Urine
30	Beta hemolytic streptotoccus	Eye
31	*P. rettgeri* (lactose ferment)	Urine
32	*C. perfringens*	Wound
33	*P. stuartii*	Leg wound
34	*P. stuartii*	Urine
35	*C. perfringens*	Chest fluid
36	*C. perfringens*	Thoracic fluid
37	*C. perfringens* with *Bacillus sp.*	Wound
38	*S. sonnei*	Urine
39	*C. perfringens* with *Bacillus sp.*	Wound
40	*P. multocida*	Wound
41	Beta hemolytic streptococcus Group A	Throat
42	*M. tuberculosis*	Sputum
43	*E. tarda*	Stool
44	*Moraxella sp.*	Eye
45	Enteropathogenic *E. coli* A	Stool
46	*S. paratyphi* A	Fluid

Figure 6-31 Blind unknowns correctly characterized.

Submitted	Reported	Error
S. Marcescens (nonpigmented) (wound)	E. aerogenes	Omission of arabinose, malonate, and gelatin.
P. stutzeri (wound)	Ps. aeruginosa	Error in interpretation of pigment. Omission of gluconate.
C. albicans (nail scrapings)	No evidence pathogenic fungi	Pseudohyphae not seen and culture omitted.
Beta hemolytic strep Group D (chest fluid)	Beta hemolytic	Reference culture in error.
E. coli (Alk-Disp) (dialysis fluid)	E. coli	False positive motility, agglutinations omitted.
Corynebacterium sp. and S. epidermidis (eye)	Nonhemolytic strep (enterococcus)	Smears of colonies not recorded. Gram positive rods ignored. Staph called strep on basis of colonial microscopic morphology.
B. anthracis (blood)	Bacillus sp.	Failure to recognize potential species and report to microbiologist.
M. polymorpha var. oxidans (urine)	Not reported	Excessive delay in identification (1 month).
Arizona sp. (urine)	Arizona	Delay caused by error in performing agglutinations (false negative).
Shigella (urine)	E. coli	Improper serological agglutination. Agglutination blocked—was not boiled.
C. perfringens (thoracentesis) P. mirabilis (chest fluid)	P. mirabilis	Gram positive rods ignored in smear of thio.
C. perfringens with P. mirabilis and Bacillus sp. (wound)	P. mirabilis Bacillus sp.	Gram positive rods in thio smear interpreted as Bacillus sp.
C. perfringens with Bacillus sp. (wound)	Bacillus sp.	Gram positive rods in thio smear interpreted as Bacillus sp.
C. perfringens (wound)	Bacteroides sp.	Gram stain overdecolorized and misinterpreted.
Clostridium sp. (wound)	E. coli P. rettgeri	Overdecolorization and contamination.
C. perfringens (chest fluid)	Sterile	Direct smear not read. Thio discarded at 48 hours. Probably inadequate planting or inoculation. Control culture grew heavily in 24 hours in thio.
Clostridium sp. (chest fluid)	Flavobacterium sp. Micrococcus sp.	Clostridium sp. recognized initially. Delay of 8 days occurred with contamination. Clostridium ignored in report.
C. perfringens (ureteral urine from cystoscopy)	Sterile	No Thio planted.
C. perfringens with Bacillus sp. (wound)	Bacillus sp.	Gram positive rods in smears interpreted as Bacillus
S. sonnei (urine)	E. coli	Unexplained gross misinterpretation of culture results and reactions.
Bacteroides, E. coli (wound), Group A beta hemolytic strep	E. coli, Group A beta hemolytic strep	Careless interpretation of Gram stains.
Bacteroides, E. coli (wound), Group A beta hemolytic strep	E. coli, Group A beta hemolytic Strep	Gram stain poor, anaerobic technique inadequate.
C. perfringens (wound), S. epidermidis	S. epidermidis	Failure to prepare Gram stain of thio that revealed Gram positive rods.
M. tuberculosis (sputum)	Acid-fast bacilli	Report requested stat but delayed 48 hours.
M. tuberculosis (sputum)	Negative	Missed on ZN, Rhodamine auramine positive.
S. paratyphi A	S. paratyphi A	Excessive delay in identification (4 days), no preliminary report.

Figure 6-32 Blind unknowns in which errors occurred.

grossly apparent numbers of cells and casts and marked disagreement in specific gravity and results of chemical tests. Many of these appear to result from the misnumbering of specimens.

It is difficult to prepare blind parasitology specimens. These must be fixed in polyvinyl alcohol or other preservatives that yield a detectable odor. Numerous other types of abnormal specimens may be preserved and resubmitted. For example, we have resubmitted a urine sample previously shown to be positive for hemosiderin with a request for a test for hemosiderin.

APPENDIX I

Surveillance Schedule
and Report

SURVEILLANCE SCHEDULE AND REPORT

An unabridged and unmodified copy of the complete Surveillance Schedule from the quality control section of the procedure manual used in our laboratory appears on pages 184–214.

The same items that appear in the Surveillance Schedule are listed in the monthly Surveillance Report which follows on pages 215–225. Technologists indicate on this report whether surveillance was conducted on schedule and whether any error was found. Portions of the Surveillance Report have been omitted to save space. For example, all media are individually listed in the actual report. This reduces the risk that failure to monitor individual media may be omitted from the report. Other portions have been modified and abbreviated.

Personnel responsible for conducting surveillance activities are defined in the Surveillance Schedule. If any item is not monitored as scheduled, an explanation must be provided on a Surveillance Report Supplement Sheet A. If any error or deficiency is found, this must be reported.

To verify that an error has been recorded on the Surveillance Report, unacceptable observations are circled on laboratory work sheets, with insertion of the letters SR, date, and initials. A complete description of the error is made on Sheet B. This must include a description of the action taken to resolve the problem, whether a solution was found, or whether the matter is pending. A and B sheets must be submitted to the supervisor for compilation into the monthly surveillance report to the Director. The supervisor reviews all "pending" deficiencies reported during the previous month. Those that continue as "pending" are submitted with the next surveillance report.

Frequency of Surveillance	I. METHODS (responsibility for surveillance is indicated under each item.)	Standards to be monitored
3 mos.	A. Procedure Book	All sections of the procedure book are indexed by author. Each section will be monitored every three months by the author. The supervisor will reassign sections when employees terminate. Corrections will be submitted to the division secretary for retyping, copying and distribution to established procedure book locations. Deficient procedures will be listed as pending until corrections are distributed.
1-6mos.	B. Evening Shift Personnel Review	Review of procedures with evening personnel by area assistant supervisor. Procedures to be reviewed and frequency will be established by supervisor.
1-6mos.	C. Night Shift Personnel Review	Review of procedures with night shift personnel by assistant supervisor. Procedures to be reviewed and frequency will be established by supervisor
1 month	D. Proficiency testing specimens	Supervisor receives samples and submits to area assistant supervisors; checks later all forms before mailing and mails before deadline. Assistant supervisor reports results at weekly meeting. Supervisor receives critique and discusses with area assistant supervisors resolving any discrepancies. Surveillance is applied to completion of analyses and mailing of reports prior to deadline; review of critiques; maintenance of specimen viability; resolution of discrepancies. To be conducted by area assistant supervisor.
1 month	E. Cultures submitted to Reference Lab.	Area assistant supervisor is responsible to: prepare and send sample to Reference Lab; copy lab slip and put in proper book; maintain sample for retest in case of discrepancies; resolution of any discrepancies; discuss results with supervisor. Surveillance is applied to resolution of discrepancies; maintenance of viability of specimens.

Frequency of Surveillance	Methods	Standards to be monitored
	I. METHODS (cont'd)	
	F. Blind Unknowns	
1 month	1. Bacteriology	In duplicate by supervisor
daily	2. Clinical Microscopy	Submitted by area assistant supervisor.
1 month	3. Serology	Submitted and results reviewed by supervisor.
2 months	4. Mycology	
1 month	5. Mycobacterium	
1 month	6. Fluorescence Microscopy	Blind unknowns are submitted by non-diagnostic supervisor. Results on all of the above are correlated and discussed with Diagnostic supervisor and area assistant supervisors. Diagnostic supervisors then discusses results.
	II. BACTERIOLOGY (Surveillance conducted by Bacteriology Asst. Supervisor)	
	A. General	
	1. Antimicrobial Susceptibility Testing Disc Method	
Each batch of medium	A. Materials	Control strains tested with each batch of media
		a. coordinate media preparation for testing
		b. coordinate stock and use of antibiotics in test
		c. maintain control strains
		d. calculate precision and error. Control reporting of results on drugs yielding unacceptable results.
3 months	B. Personnel	Test each worker for technique, precision and accuracy every three months.
Monthly or as requested	2. Antimicrobial Susceptibility Testing-tube dilution-Penicillin	Monitor technique and procedure with stock strain of Enterococcus of know MIC. Results must be 3-12 units/ml
	B. Biologicals, Frequently Used	
6 mos	1. Antisera for bacteriologic identification E. coli, A,B,C, H. influenzae, A & B	Culture antisera in use 6 months-rotate all antisera in use, according to inventory. Test new antisera with known cultures.

Frequency of Surveillance	Item	Standards to be monitored
	II. Bacteriology (cont'd)	
	B. Biologicals (cont.)	
Each use	Shigella A-D Salmonella A-I, vi, polyvalent Alkalescens dispar Bathesda Ballerup Arizona * a. Check specificity with homologous cultures b. Check for sterility	* Test homologous bacterial culture.
	1. Stains	
Monthly	Gram stain reagents	Fresh stock dated. Discard remaining portions every 6 months.
Monthly	Flagella stain	Fresh stock dated. Discard remaining portions yearly. Combined stain made fresh with each use and discarded after use.
Monthly	Hydrogen Peroxide	Replace with Fresh Stock every two months.
	C. Equipment (Surveillance to be conducted by assistant supervisor in each area)	Standard
	1. Refrigerators	
Weekly	MB 4338-Foster 2 door	2-8°C
	4348 Jewett	2-8°C
	4347 Foster 6 door	2-8°C
	Foster 5 door	2-8°C
6 months		Test automatic alarms
	2. Freezer	
Weekly	MB 4307 Dillon Lilly	-8°C
	3. Incubators	
	MB 4339 Labline 1d	
	MB 4371 Labline 2d	
Weekly	temperatures	
Weekly	water	
Weekly	Fan motors	pan full running smoothly
6 months	Vents	MB4371 oil with 20 SAE
6 months		change glasswool filter

C. Equipment (cont'd)

3. Incubators (cont.)

MB 4380 Labline CO_2

Item	Frequency	Standard
temperature	Weekly	$35 \pm 1\,^\circ C$
water	Weekly	Bubbler system full
fans	Weekly	running smoothly
fan motor	6 months	oil with 20 SAE
CO_2 tanks	Weekly	tanks not empty
surge tank	Weekly	12 lbs. during surge
flow tank	Weekly	12 lbs at .3 LPM
CO_2 concentration	Yearly	5-10%
		Monitor for 48 hrs with medical gas analyzer (Pulmonary Lab)
		Syringe full of gas
Humidity	Monthly	60-80%
	Weekly	

4. Water baths and Heating Blocs

Item	Frequency	Standard
MB Hospital Control	Weekly	$54-56\,^\circ C$
MB 4319 variable	Weekly	
MB 4369 TSN bloc	Weekly	$45-47\,^\circ C$
MB 4368 variable	Weekly	

Item	Frequency	Standard
5. Inoculating Loops	Monthly	3mm diam. replace as needed
6. Inoculating wire	Monthly	5-8cm, replace as needed
7. Safety Hood	6 months	Face velocity 50 rpm
	Monthly	Filter pressure 0.5-1.5cm
	3 months	Wash interior with germicidal cleaner
8. Air Conditioner Rm 336	Monthly	Change filter (by Engineering)
9. Grinding motor	6 months	oiled
	6 months	fan belt, wear, tension
10. Microscopes	Monthly	General inspection

C. Equipment (cont'd)

Frequency of Surveillance		Standard
Daily Daily Daily	11. Anaerobic jars	Clost. novyii control Change catalyst Anaerobic indicator

III. Immunology (surveillance to be conducted by area assistant supervisor)

A. Procedures

Frequency of Surveillance		Standards to be monitored
As performed or once a month	1. Antistreptolysis "O" titer 2. Brucella 3. Rheumatoid Factor 4. Thyroglobulin antibody 5. Typhoid O 6. VDRL 7. Antinuclear Factor 8. E. coli 9. N. gonorrhoeae 10. Strep 11. Rhodamine -Auramine staining of mycobacteria	Prepare and distribute positive and negative controls, approve results before reporting. Record control data graphically
Weekly	12. VDRL	Monitor proper use and recording of controls Graphically record comparison of State Lab and Hartford Hospital results. Resolve results differing by more than two tubes.
Monthly	13. Rhodamine-auramine stain	Fresh stock dated. Discard remaining portion every two months.

B. Equipment

Frequency of Surveillance		Standard
Weekly. Test automatic alarms each 6 months.	1. Refrigerators MB 4357	2-8 °C
Weekly	2. Waterbaths MB 4384 VDRL MB 4390 Misc. 3. VDRL Rotators MB 4335 F.A. MB 4387 VDRL	55-57 °C 36-38°C Lubricate bearings Check brushes

Standard

B. Equipment (cont'd)

3. VDRL Rotators — 180 rpm (VDRL only) — Weekly

4. Inoculating loops — 5 mm. diam. loop — Replace monthly or as needed

5. Safety Hood — Face velocity 50-200 FPM — 6 months

6. Microscopes — General inspection — 6 months

7. Fluorolume Illuminator 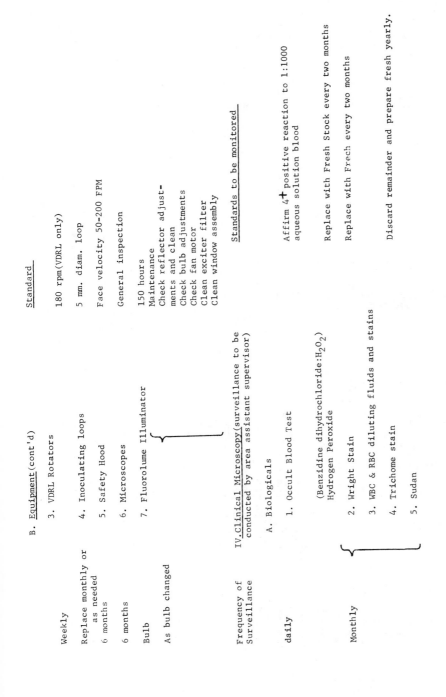 — 150 hours
Maintenance
Check reflector adjust-
ments and clean
Check bulb adjustments
Check fan motor
Clean exciter filter
Clean window assembly
— Bulb / As bulb changed

IV. Clinical Microscopy (surveillance to be conducted by area assistant supervisor)

Frequency of Surveillance

Standards to be monitored

A. Biologicals

1. Occult Blood Test — Affirm 4+ positive reaction to 1:1000 aqueous solution blood — daily

(Benzidine dihydrochloride:H_2O_2)
Hydrogen Peroxide

2. Wright Stain — Replace with Fresh Stock every two months — Monthly

3. WBC & RBC diluting fluids and stains — Replace with Fresh every two months

4. Trichome stain

5. Sudan — Discard remainder and prepare fresh yearly.

189

IV. Clinical Microscopy (cont'd)

B. Equipment

Frequency	Equipment	Standard
Weekly	1. Refrigerator MB 4372	2-8 $^\circ$C
6 months		Test automatic alarms
3 months	2. Refractometer MB 4388 MB 4390	Calibrate with H_2O to 1.000
Discard monthly as found	3. Glassware	Chipped
3 months	4. Fume Hood	Wash with germicidal cleaner
Monthly	5. Microscopes	General Inspection

V. Media Room (surveillance to be conducted by media room personnel)

A. Equipment

Frequency	Equipment	Standard
Weekly	1. Refrigerator MB 4394	2-8 $^\circ$C
Daily	2. Hot Air Oven	Record each run; must be 155-165 $^\circ$C
3 months		Sterility check (spore strips)
3 months	3. Autoclaves	Sterility check (spore solution)
Weekly		Check gaskets
Monthly	4. Glassware	Discard chipped glassware
3 months	5. Balance	Calibrate
6 months		Clean and general maintenance (described in instruction manual)

VI. <u>Mycology</u> (Surveillance to be conducted by area assistant supervisor)   <u>Standard</u>

A. <u>Equipment</u>

Weekly	1. Waterbaths	
Weekly	2. Incubator MB 4350	35 ± 1 C
6 months	3. Safety Hood	Face velocity 50-200fpm
3 months		Wash with germicidal cleaner
Monthly	4. Microscope	General Inspection

VII. <u>Miscellaneous</u> (surveillance to be conducted by delegated supervisor)

A. <u>Equipment</u>

	1. Vacuum pump-Precision Scientific (for lyophilization)	Before use and when in continual use the following are performed
3 months		$\frac{1}{2}$" belt tension
3 months		oil level
6 months		oil parts
Yearly		change oil, order new oil
6 months	2. Vacuum pump-Gomco Surgical Pump	oil as indicated
As received	3. Pipettes	Calibrate representative
As received	4. Thermometers	Calibrate with NBS calibrated thermometer

191

VIII <u>Media Surveillance</u> (Surveillance functions to be delegated by supervisor)

Item	Standard to be monitored		Frequency
A. Autoclave cycles	Recording of minutes of exposure to 121°C		
	Min.	Max.	
1. Test tubes 18 x 150mm with 10ml agar	12	34	Every batch
2. 1000ml volume in flask	20	54	Every batch
3. 2000ml volume in flask	30	72	Every batch
B. pH	Must be $\pm$0.2 from recommended pH of manufacturer (except Mueller-Hinton 7.2-7.4)		Every Batch

C. Storage	Conditions	Duration	
1. Plates	2-8°C		
	Not bagged	2 weeks	
	Bagged	8 weeks	
2. Tubes	2-8°C		Weekly
	Sponge-plug		
	Not bagged	2 weeks	
	Bagged	2 months	
	Screw-capped		
	No bagged	2 months	
	Bagged	4 months	

3. Exceptions noted with individual items below

a. CTA sugars Room temperature 2 weeks

b. Indole Nitrate Room temperature 2 weeks In plastic bags

c. Thioglycollate Room temperature 2 weeks Dark

Media Surveillance (cont)

Item	Standard to be monitored	Frequency
D. Depth of plates		
1. plates	3mm(except Mueller-Hinton 4-6mm)	Every Batch
2. Tubes		
a. agar	length of slant equal to length of butt	
b. broths	specified in reagents and media section	
E. Sterility Check		
1. Broth	3 tubes incubated 48 hours	Each Batch
2. Plates	5% of plates incubated 48 hours (chocolate agar 72 hours and omit MacConkey)	Each Batch
F. Testing of Stock Cultures	Proper hemolysis Correct color reactions Inhibitory or selective properties 24 hour incubation	Each batch* or each lot +

Item	Control Organisms	Acceptable Results
A. BAP*	Group A beta-hemolytic Strep Strep viridans Blank	Good beta-hemolysis Good alpha-hemolysis Sterile
B. Biplates*	See BAP and Mac	See BAP and Mac
C. Brain Heart* Infusion agar	Cryptococcus sp.	Growth
D. Brain Heart* Infusion agar and Chloramphenicol	Nocardia sp. E. coli	Growth No growth
E. Casein plates*	Streptomyces sp. Nocardia asteroides	Hydrolysis No hydrolysis

193

Media Surveillance (cont)

F. Testing of Stock Cultures

	Control Organisms	Acceptable Results
F. Chocolate*	Hemophilus influenzae	Good growth
	Neisseria gonorrhoeae	Good growth (48 hours)
G. Martin-Lester	Neisseria gonorrhoea	Good growth (48 hours)
	Staph aureus	Inhibition
	E. coli	Inhibition
	Proteus mirabilis	Inhibition of swarming
	Candida albicans	Inhibition
H. MacConkey+	E. coli	Lactose pos;correct morphology
	Shigella flexneri (B)	colorless colonies
	Enterococcus	Inhibition
I. Mycobiotic Agar*	Candida albicans	Growth
	Aspergillus	No growth
	E. coli	No growth
J. Mueller-Hinton*	See surveillance of disk susceptibility test section II,A,1	Disc
K. PEA*	Staph aureus	Growth
	E. coli	Inhibition(tiny colonies)
	Pseudomonas aeruginosa	Inhibition(tiny colonies)
L. Potato Dextrose Agar*	T. rubrum	Growth
M. Rice Agar*	Candida albicans	Chlamydospores (72 hours)
	Candida krusei	No chlamydospores(72 hours)
N. Rodac*	Flavobacterium	Growth
O. Sabouraud's Dextrose*	Candida albicans	Growth
P. Sabouraud's Dextrose* Agar & Chloramphenicol	Aspergillus sp.	Growth
	E. coli	No growth
Q. Trypticase Soy Agar+	Staph aureus	Growth
	Strep viridans	Growth
R. Tyrosine plates*	Streptomyces sp.	Positive
	Nocardia asteroides	Negative

Media Surveillance (cont)

F. Testing of Stock Cultures

	Control Organisms	Acceptable Results
S. Xanthine plates*	Streptomyces sp. Nocardia asteroides	Positive Negative
T. XLD	Salmonella typhimurium Shigella flexneri (B) E. coli	black colonies red(colorless) colonies yellow colonies

G. Testing of Tubed Media with stock cultures

	Control Organisms	Acceptable Results
1. Christensen's urea*	Proteus mirabilis Klebsiella pneumoniae E. coli	+ D 0
2. Christensen's urea*slants (mycology version)	Torulopsis sp. Candida sp.	Positive Negative
3. DNase*	Serratia Staph epidermidis	+ 0
4. Middlebrook 7H-10*	Nocardia Mycobacterium tuberculosis	Positive Positive
5. Pseudosel*	Pseudomonas aeruginosa E. coli	Growth and pigment + + 0 0

	Control Organisms	H_2S	indol	motility
6. Sim+	Proteus mirabilis	+	0	+
	Klebsiella pneumoniae	0	+	+
	E. coli	0	+	+

	Control Organisms	Acceptable Results
7. Simmon's citrate+	Klebsiella pneumoniae E. coli	+ 0
8. Stuart's Transport+	Neiserria gonorrhoeae 22°C 6 hour transfer 2-8°C 6 hour transfer	Growth 48 hours Growth 48 hours
	Clostridium novyii 22°C 6 hour transfer 2-8°C 6 hour transfer	Growth 24 hours Growth 24 hours

Media Surveillance (cont).

G. Testing of Tubed Media with stock cultures

	Control Organisms	Acceptable Results
9. TSA+	Staph aureus	Growth
	Strep viridans	Growth
10. TSI+	E. coli	A/AG
	Salmonella typhimurium	ALK/AG H$_2$S+
	Proteus rettgeri	ALK/A
	Pseudomonas aeruginosa	ALK/NC
11. TSN+	Clostridium perfringens	+
	Clostridium novyii	0

Semi-solids

12. OF sugars*

	Prot. rettgeri Lactose ferm.	Proteus morgani	Pseudomonas aeruginosa	Pseudomonas maltophilia	Arizona
a. glucose	A	A	A/O	0	A
b. sucrose	A	0	0	0	0
c. maltose	0	0	0	A	A
d. lactose	A	0	0	0	A
e. xylose	0	0	A	0	A
f. arabinose	Serratia Enterobacter	A			

13. CTA sugars*

	Neisseria gonorrhoeae	Neisseris meningitidis	Neisseria sicca		Neisseria catarrhalis
a. glucose	A	A	A		0
b. maltose	0	A	A		0
c. sucrose	0	0	A		0
d. lactose	0	0	0		0

Media Surveillance (cont)

Semi solids	Control Organisms	Acceptable Results
14. Indole Nitrate*	Indole	
	E. coli	+
	Klebsiella pneumoniae	0
	Nitrate	
	Staph aureus	+
	Herellea sp.	0
	Pseudomonas aeruginosa	+ g
15. Gelatin*(mycology version)	Cladosporium	Positive
	F. pedrosoi	Negative
16. Rice Grains*	M. canis	Positive
	M. audouini	Negative
17. Bile*(Na desoxycholate)	D. pneumoniae	+
	Strep viridans	0
18. Blood Broth*	Hemophilus influenzae	Growth 24 hours
	Neisseria meningitidis	Growth 24 hours
19. Brain Heart Infusion*	Cryptococcus albidus	Growth
20. Brain Heart Insusion & Chloramphenicol*	Cryptococcus albidus	Growth
21. Decarboxylase*		
a. Control*	Proteus mirabilis	0
	Klebsiella pneumoniae	0
	Pseudomonas aeruginosa	NC
b. with ornithine*	Proteus mirabilis	+
	Klebsiella pneumoniae	0
	Pseudomonas aeruginosa	NC
c. with lysine*	E. coli	+
	Enterobacter cloacae	0
	Pseudomonas aeruginosa	NC
22. Gelatin*	Pseudomonas aeruginosa	+
	Herellea	0

Media Surveillance (cont)

Item	Control Organisms	Acceptable Results
23. Gluconate+	Pseudomonas aeruginosa	+
	Herellea	0
24. G-N Broth +	E. coli:Shigella=1:1	
	6 hour transfer	recovery of Shigella
	18 hour transfer	recovery of Shigella inhibition of E. coli
	E. coli:Shigella=2:1	
	6 hour transfer	recovery of Shigella
	18 hour transfer	recovery of Shigella
25. Inositol*	Trichosporon verrucosum	Positive
26. Malonate +	Klebsiella pneumoniae	+
	E. coli	0
27. MRVP +	E. coli	+/0
	Klebsiella pneumoniae	0/+
28. ONPG +	E. coli	+
	Proteus mirabilis	0
29. PAD*	Proteus mirabilis	+
	E. coli	0
30. PSE +	Enterococcus	+
	Group D not Enterococcus	+
	Listeria (48 hours)	+
	Group A beta-hemolytic Strep	0
31. Rabbit Plasma +	Staph aureus	+
	Staph epidermidis	0
32. 6.5% salt broth *	Enterococcus	+
	Group D not Enterococcus	0
	Staph aureus	+
	Group A beta-hemolytic Strep	0
33. Sucrose assimilation*	Candida albicans	+

198

Media Surveillance (cont)

Item	Control Organisms	Acceptable Results
34. Thiamine*	T. tonsurans T. menta	+ 0
35. Thioglycollate +	Clostridium novyii Strep viridans	Growth Growth
36. Trypticase Soy Broth+	Strep viridans	Growth-24 hours
37. Urea broth*(Rustigian & Stewart)	N. brasiliens	+

IX Inventory of reagents and biologicals

Storage Code

A-Room temperature

B-2-8°

C-Cool

D-Dry

E-Protect from light

F-Dangerous to handle for one or more of the following:

1. Poison

2. Caustic

3. Corrosive

4. Avoid contact (absorbed through skin, strong ixidizing agent, etc.)

5. Should not be inhaled

6. Volatile

7. Extremely toxic

8. Carcinogen

G-Freeze

H-Dessicated

NS-None stated or none found in reference

Expiration Code

M-Month

W-Week

Y-Year

Expiration Code(cont)

S-Stated on product

D-Does not apply

NS-None stated or none found in references

References

Merck Index of Chemical and Drugs, Merck & Co., Rahway, New Jersey 1960

BBL Manual of Products and Laboratory Procedures, Bioquest, Cockeysville, Maryland,5th Edition,1968

Personal Communication, David A. Power, Ph.D., Director, Technical Services,BBL

A) Biologicals-Immunology(Surveillance to be conducted by area assistant supervisor)

Item	Expiration Date opened	closed	Storage opened	closed	Surveillance interval
Albumin, Bovine	2M	3Y	B	B	Weekly
ANF conjugate	6M	1y	G	B	Weekly
ASO Buffer	1M	2Y or S	B	B	Weekly
ASO Reagent	10 min.	2Y or S	B	B	Weekly
ASO Standard	2M	2Y or S	G	B	Weekly
Brucella	2M	S	B	B	Weekly
E. coli A-conjugate(Difco)	2M	1Y	B	B	Weekly
E. coli A-serological	6M	2Y	B	B	Weekly
E. coli B-conjugate (Difco)	2M	1Y	B	B	Weekly
E. coli B-serological	6M	2Y	B	B	Weekly
E. coli C-conjugate	2M	1Y	B	B	Weekly
E. coli C-serological	6M	2Y	B	B	Weekly
Typhoid "O" and Brucella control-neg.	3M	NS	G	B	Weekly
Typhoid "O" and Brucella control-pos.	3M	S	G	B	Weekly
Hemagglutination Buffer	1M	2Y	B	B	Weekly
Monospot Kit	1M	S	B	B	Weekly
Neisseria gonorrhoeae conjugate	2M	1Y	B	B	Weekly
PBS (Phospate Buffered Saline)	1M	NS	B	A	Weekly
Pregnosticon-(slide) 50 test	2W	S	B	B	Weekly
10 test	1M	S	B	B	Weekly
Pregnosticon-Accusphere		S	B	B	Weekly
R A Buffer	1M	S	B	B	Weekly

A) Biologicals (cont) - Immunology

Item	Expiration Date		Storage		Surveillance
	opened	closed	opened	closed	Interval
R. A. Latex 0.81	1M	1Y	B	B	Weekly
R A Plasma Fraction II	1M	1Y	B	B	Weekly
R A Test Kit	1M	S	B	B	Weekly
Rabbit Globulin-FITC labelled F.A.	2M	1Y	B	B	Weekly
Rabbit Plasma,normal-FA discard remainder after use	2W	1Y	B	B	Weekly
Strep conjugate *	2M	4M			Weekly
	Depends on manufacturer				
*Strep Controls					
positrol	2M	1Y	A	B	Weekly
negatrol	2M	1Y	A	B	Weekly
Streptozyme kit	1M	S	B	B	Weekly
VDRL control sera	3M	S	G	B	Weekly
Thyroid kit	1M	S	B	B	Weekly
Typhoid "O"	2W	S	B	B	Weekly
VDRL antigen and buffer	2W	1Y	A	E	Weekly

B) Biologicals-Bacteriology(Surveillance to be conducted by area assistant supervisor)

Item	Expiration Date		Storage		Surveillance
	opened	closed	opened	closed	Interval
Ampicillin	6M	S	GH	GH	Weekly
Arizona diphasic	1Y	S	B	B	Weekly
Arizona monophasic Open when needed	1Y	S	B	B	Weekly
Carbenicillin	6M	S	GH	GH	Weekly

B) Biologicals-Bacteriology(cont)

Item	Expiration Date opened	closed	Storage opened	closed	Surveillance Interval
Cephalothin	6M	S	GH	BH	Weekly
Chloramphenicol	6M	S	GH	BH	Weekly
Colistin	6M	S	GH	BH	Weekly
Erythromycin	6M	S	GH	BH	Weekly
Gentamicin sulfate	6M	S	GH	BH	Weekly
Hemophilus Type A	6M	S	B	B	Weekly
Hemophilus type B	6M	S	B	B	Weekly
Horse Serum	6M	1Y	0-4° C	0-4° C	Monthly
Kanamycin	6M	S	GH	BH	Weekly
Lincomycin hydrochloride	6M	S	GH	BH	Weekly
Methicillin	6M	S	GH	GH	Weekly
Naladixic acid	6M	S	BH	BH	Weekly
Nitrofurantoin	6M	S	BH	BH	Weekly
Omni serum for pneumococcus	1Y	2Y	0-5° C	0-5° C	Weekly
Oxytetracycline	6M	S	GH	BH	Weekly
Penicillin-disc	6M	S	GH	GH	Weekly
Penicillin-powder,standard	6M	S	GH	GH	Weekly
Penicillinase	1Y	5Y	B	B	Weekly
Rabbit plasma,normal-coag.	2W	3Y	G	B	Weekly
Salmonella O Group A	6M	2Y	B	B	Weekly
Salmonella O Group B	6M	2Y	B	B	Weekly

B) Biologicals-Bacteriology (cont)

Item	Expiration Date Opened	Expiration Date Closed	Storage Opened	Storage Closed	Surveillance Interval
Salmonella O Group C1	6M	2Y	B	B	Weekly
Salmonella O Group C2	6M	2Y	B	B	Weekly
Salmonella O Group D	6M	2Y	B	B	Weekly
Salmonella O Group E	6M	2Y	B	B	Weekly
Salmonella O Group F	6M	2Y	B	B	Weekly
Salmonella O Group G	6M	2Y	B	B	Weekly
Salmonella O Group H	6M	2Y	B	B	Weekly
Salmonella O Group I	6M	2Y	B	B	Weekly
Salmonella O polyvalent	6M	1Y	B	B	Weekly
Salmonella Vi	6M	2Y	B	B	Weekly
Shigella Group A	6M	2Y	B	B	Weekly
Shigella Group B	6M	2Y	B	B	Weekly
Shigella Group C	6M	2Y	B	B	Weekly
Shigella Group D	6M	2Y	B	B	Weekly
Shigella-Alkalescens-dispar	6M	2Y	B	B	Weekly
Streptomycin	6M	S	GH	BH	Weekly
Sulfisoxizol(Gantrisin)	6M	S	BH	BH	Weekly
Tetracycline	6M	S	GH	BH	Weekly
Vancomycin hydrochloride	6M	S	BH	BH	Weekly

Stock Carbohydrates	Surveillance	Expiration date opened	closed	Storage	Frequency of surveillance
Frequently used stored in crystal form					
Arabinose					
Dextrose					
Lactose		6M	2Y	CD	Weekly
Maltose					
Sucrose					
D-xylose					
Infrequently used stored in taxo disc form					
Adonitol					
Dulcitol					
Galactose					
Inositol					
Inulin					
Levulose		6M	2Y	BH	Monthly
Mannitol					
Mannose					
Raffinose					
Rhamnose					
Salicin					
Sorbitol					
Trehalose					

Stock Chemicals	Storage and/or Precautions	Expiration	Frequency of Surveillance
Acetic acid, Glacial	F_1, 4	N.S.	M
N-acetyl L-cysteine	B_1	N.S.	M
Auramine O	D	5Y	M
p-Aminodimethylaniline ozalate	D	N.S.	M
Ammonium Sulfate Powder		N.S.	M
Aniline	F_1E	N.S.	M
Barium Chloride	F_1	N.S.	M
Barium sulfate	N.S.	3M prepared	M
Benzidine Dihydrochloride	N.S.	6M prepared	M
Brom thymol Blue		5Y	M
Calcium Chloride	C,D	N.S.	M
China Blue Powder(Poirrier's Blue)	D	N.S.	M
Chlorazol Black E	D	5Y	M
Crystal Violet	D	5Y	M
Cysteine hydrochloride	D	N.S.	M
p-Dimethylaminobenzaldyhde	E	N.S.	M
Dimethylsulfoxide	N.S.	N.S.	M
Eosin Y	D	5Y	M
Ether	F5,6		M
Ethyl Alcohol	D	3M opened N.S. sealed	

Stock Chemicals	Storage and/or Precautions	Expiration	Frequency of Surveillance
Ferric Ammonium Citrate	E	N.S.	M
Ferric Chloride	E	N.S.	M
Fuchsin Acid	D	5Y	M
Fuchsin,Basic	D	5Y	M
Glycerine	F4	N.S.	M
Gramercy Indicator	N.S.	N.S.	M
Hemin	N.S.	N.S.	M
Hcl,conc. Chemistry	F4,5	N.S.	M
Hydrogen Peroxide 3%	E,C,F2	N.S.	M
Iodine Crystals	N.S.	N.S.	M
Lactic Acid	N.S.	N.S.	M
Magnesium sulfate	D	N.S.	M
Malachite Green	D	5Y	M
Menadione	E	N.S.	M
Mercuric Chloride	F 1	N.S.	M
Merthiolate		N.S.	M
Methylene Blue	D,F 1	5Y	M
Methyl Red	D	5Y	M
Monosodium and Citric Acid			
Naphthol	E	N.S.	M
Naphythylamine	F4	N.S.	M
Orthonitrophenyl-B-d-Galactopyranoside	N.S.	N.S.	M

Stock Chemicals	Storage and/or Precautions	Expiration	Frequency of Surveillance
Oxgall	C,D	1Y opened	M
Periodic Acid	N.S.	N.S.	M
Phenol(crystals)	D,E,F$_4$	N.S.	M
Phenophthalein diphosphate	F4	N.S.	M
Phenyl Red	D	5Y	M
Phenylalanine	N.S.	N.S.	M
Potassium Alum	N.S.	N.S.	M
Potassium ferrocyanide	N.S.	working sol.-immediately	M
Potassium Hydroxide	F$_2$	N.S.	M
Potassium Iodide	N.S.	N.S.	M
Potassium Permanganate	D	5Y	M
Potassium Phosphate Dibasic	N.S.	N.S.	M
Potassium Phosphate Monobasic	N.S.	N.S.	M
Rhodamine O	D,F$_1$	5Y	M
Safranin	D	5Y	M
Sedi stain	D	5Y	M
Sodium carbonate	D,E,F 1,4	N.S.	M
Sodium Chloride	N.S.	N.S.	M
Sodium Citrate	N.S.	N.S.	M
Sodium Desoxycholate	N.S.	N.S.	M
Sodium Hydroxide	F$_2$	N.S.	M

Stock Chemicals	Storage and/or Precautions	Expiration	Frequency of Surveillance
Sodium meta bisulfate	N.S.	N.S.	M
Sodium Phosphate Monobasic	N.S.	N.S.	M
Sodium Phosphate Tribasic	N.S.	N.S.	M
Sodium Succinate	N.S.	N.S.	M
Sodium Thiosulfate	N.S.	N.S.	M
Sudan III	D	5Y	M
Sulfanilic Acid	N.S.	N.S.	M
Sulfosalicylic Acid	D,E	N.S.	M
Tannic Acid	E	N.S.	M
N,N,N, Tetrametyl-p-phenylene diamine monohydrochloride	F_1,4	N.S.	M
Thiamine	N.S.	N.S.	M
Thymol-merck	N.S.	N.S.	M
Toluidine Blue	D,F_1	5Y	M
Trichome	D	5Y	M
Trisodium Citrate			M
Triphenyltetrazolium Chloride	N.S.	N.S.	M
Trypan Blue	D	5Y	M
L-tryptophane	N.S.	N.S.	M
Tyrosine	N.S.	N.S.	M
Xanthine	F_1	N.S.	M

Stock Chemicals		Storage and/or Precautions		Frequency of Surveillance
Zinc sulfate		F_5	N.S.	M
Zinc Dust Metal				

C) Media (Surveillance to be conducted by Media Room personnel under direction of Supervisor)

Product	Dept.	Expiration Date opened	closed	Storage
AGAR Agar	B	1Y	3Y	CD
Anaerobic Agar	B	1Y	3Y	CD
Brain Heart Infusion Agar	B	1Y	3Y	CD
Brain Heart Infusion Broth	A	1Y	3Y	CD
Brilliant Green Agar	B	1Y	3Y	CD
Bordet Gengou	B	1Y	3Y	CD
Chloramphenicol	A	6M	S	B.D.
Columbia Agar Base	B	1Y	3Y	CD
Clostrisel Agar	B	1Y	2Y	CD
Cooked Meat Medium	B	1Y	3Y	CD
CTA Medium	B	1Y	3Y	CD
DNase Test Medium	B	1Y	3Y	CD
Entamoeba Medium	B	1Y	3Y	CD
Fletcher Medium Base	B	1Y	3Y	CD
G.C.Medium Base	B	1Y	3Y	CD
Gelatin	A	1Y	3Y	CD
G.N. Broth	B	1Y	3Y	CD

C)Media(cont)

Product	Dept.	Expiration Date		Storage
		opened	closed	
Indole Nitrate Broth	B	1Y	3Y	CD
Litmus Milk	B	1Y	2Y	CD
Loeffler Blood serum	B	1Y	2Y	CD
Lysine Iron Agar	B	1Y	2Y	CD
Mueller Hinton Agar	B	1Y	3Y	CD
Malonate	B	1Y	3Y	CD
Moeller Decarboxylase	B	1Y	3Y	B
MRVP	B	1Y	3Y	CD
Mycobiotic	B	1Y	2Y	CD
MacConkey	B	1Y	3Y	CD
Neopeptone	B	1Y	3Y	CD
OF Basal Medium	B	1Y	3Y	CD
PEA	B	1Y	3Y	B
Phenol Red Broth Base	B	1Y	3Y	CD
Phytone Peptone	A	1Y	3Y	CD
Plate Count Agar	B	1Y	3Y	CD
Pseudosel	B	1Y	3Y	CD
Purple Milk	B	1Y	3Y	CD
Resazurin	A	1Y	3Y	CD
Rice Extract Agar	B	1Y	3Y	CD
Sabaroud Agar.Modified	B	1Y	3Y	CD

C) Media (cont)

Product	Dept.	Expiration Date		Storage
		opened	closed	
SF Medium	B	1Y	3Y	CD
Skim Milk Powder	A	1Y	3Y	
SIM	B	1Y	3Y	CD
Simmons Citrate	B	1Y	3Y	CD
Spirit Blue Agar	B	1Y	3Y	CD
Stuarts Transport	B	1Y	3Y	B
Tellurite Glycine Agar Base	B	1Y	3Y	CD
TB Niacin Test	B	1Y	1Y	CD
TCBS Medium				
Thiogel Medium	B	1Y	3Y	CD
Thioglycollate with Dextrose and EH indicator	B	1Y	3Y	CD
Thioglycollate without Dextrose and EH indicator	B	1Y	3Y	CD
Todd Hewitt	B	1Y	3Y	CD
Trypticase Soy Agar with Lethicin and Polysorbate 80	B	1Y	3Y	B
Trypticase Soy Agar	B	1Y	3Y	B
Trypticase Soy Broth	B	1Y	3Y	CD
Thioglycollate Fluid	B	1Y	3Y	CD
TSI	B	1Y	3Y	CD
TSN	B	1Y	2Y	CD

C)Media (cont)

| Product | Dept. | Expiration Date | | Storage |
		opened	closed	
Urea Agar Base	B	1Y	2Y	B
Urea Broth	M	1Y		
XL Agar Base	B	1Y	2Y	CD
Yeast Extract	B	1Y	3Y	CD
Mycobactosel Agar	B	D	1Y	B
Littman Oxgall(prepared)	B	D	S	B
Loeffler(Prepared)	B	D	1Y	B
Mycobactosel L-J Agar	B	D	1Y	B

Reports that follow the Surveillance Report provide a complete description of omission of surveillance, errors that are detected, and action that is taken to resolve omission and error.

The monthly report data provided here cover the month of December 1972 and include reports of errors depicted in Figures 6-5, 6-6, 6-9, 6-14, 6-18, 6-21, 6-23, and 6-30.

Surveillance Report

Quality Control Program
Division of Microbiology
Department of Pathology
Hartford Hospital

For period __12|1|72 – 12|31|72__

Submitted __1|2|73__

Describe any items in category   Describe any deficiencies as
not conducted as scheduled   observed in category

*List page of A or B explanatory sheet

	Conducted as scheduled		Deficiencies observed	
	Yes	No*	Yes*	No
I. Methods				
A. Procedure Book	✓	-----	-----	✓
B. Evening Shift Review	✓	------	-----	✓
C. Night Shift Review	-----	1	2	-----
D. Proficiency Test Specimens	✓	------	-----	✓
E. Reference Specimens	✓	------	3	-----
F. Blind Unknowns	✓	------	4	-----
II. Bacteriology				
A. Susceptibility Test				
1. Disk				
a. materials	✓	------	5	------
b. personnel	✓	------	6	------
2. Tube Dilution	✓	------	-----	✓
B. Biological materials				
1. Antisera	✓	------	-----	✓
2. Stains	✓	------	-----	✓
C. Equipment				
1. Refrigerators	✓	------	7	------
III. Immunology				
A. Procedures	✓	------	8-9	------
VII. Media	✓	------	10	------

Use for each surveillance item not conducted as scheduled. Use
additional sheets if necessary.

ITEM _Night Shift Review_

Reason not conducted:

_Have not been able to get John Smith
to come in for scheduled review. Have
rescheduled it twice_
MP 12/5/72

Action taken:

_Discussed with Dr. Bartlett who called
him and told him he would not be
scheduled for duty until review was
conducted_
MP 12/7/72

Figure AI-1 Surveillance Report Supplement Sheet A used to explain the omission of a surveillance measure (in this case involving nightshift workers) and corrective action to be taken.

SHEET B

Use for items when surveillance reveals deficiency.

ITEM _Night Shift Review_____ _Jack Jones_____

Deficiency observed: Date_ 12/15/72 _____

Describe:

Planted sputum for anaerobic culture
Scored quality of sputum incorrectly
Forgot to initial slip

Date corrective action taken__ 12/16/72 _____

Nature of corrective action:

Reviewed lower respiratory procedures with him
Reminded to report sputums for anaerobic culture
with request for tracheobronchial secretions for
anaerobic culture. Jones said he had not
handled sputums recently at night and would
reread procedure. Repeat in 3 months

Was deficiency corrected?   ____YES   ✓ NO   Date 12/16/72

If not corrected EXPLAIN

Must await review in 3 months

Further surveillance needed (✓)   AS

Figure AI-2 Surveillance Report Supplement Sheet B used to provide an explanation of observed deficiency; in this case a review of procedures with a night worker (see Figure 6-5, p. 135).

SHEET B

Use for items when surveillance reveals deficiency.

ITEM _Ref lab Culture   HH 320_

Deficiency observed: Date ___12/17/72___

Describe:

1) Error in speciation – N. subflava called N. meningitidis. Resulted from failure to grow at 22°C. Pigmentation not noted on slip
2) Delays – no preliminary report sent. Final report 5 days. Two weeks delay in sending to reference lab

Date corrective action taken ___12/17/72___

Nature of corrective action:

Discussed with technician. Repeated 22°C culture – positive when temp controlled. Must find way to control temp – culture was put on cold window sill. Also should have repeated it if speciation depends on it. Should have studied pigment more carefully. Delays reviewed also

Was deficiency corrected: ___YES ___NO Date 12/20/72

If not corrected EXPLAIN

No control over "room temperature". Further surveillance needed for delays in handling

JT

Further surveillance needed (✓)

Figure AI-3 Report of discrepancies observed in a comparison of results with those obtained by a reference laboratory (see Figure 6-6, p. 138).

SHEET B

Use for items when surveillance reveals deficiency.

ITEM _Blind Unknown_____

Deficiency observed: Date___12/27/72_____

Describe:

Correctly identified as E. coli but other
errors made. Motility called positive. A-D
antisera not used, no preliminary report was
sent and final report was delayed 12
days. Streptomycin zone was incorrectly
interpreted

Date corrective action taken___12/27/72_____

Nature of corrective action:

Repeated discrepant tests — confirmed stock
card results — discussed errors and delays
with technician

_____

_____

_____

Was deficiency corrected?   _____YES   __✓__NO Date 12/27/72 —

If not corrected EXPLAIN

Further surveillance needed (✓/   Signed __HB_____

Figure AI-4 Report of discrepancies observed in processing a blind unknown culture (see Figure 6-30, p. 177).

ITEM	DATE OBSERVED	OBSERVATION	DATE ACTION TAKEN	ACTION TAKEN	RESULTS OF ACTION TAKEN	PROCEDURE CHANGES
Susc Test Controls (Disk test)	12/3	Ceph and Poly too large	12/3	Susc not reported		
	12/6	Strep and Tetra too large	12/6	Susc not reported		
	12/10	Colistin too large	12/10	Susc not reported		None
	12/15	Chlor and Meth too small	12/15	Resistance not reported		
	12/31	Tet too large	12/31	Susc not reported		
				No consistent error. Colistin zones larger on MH-34 than MH-39 — use MH-34. BaSO4 checked OK	Colistin zones larger MH-34	
					JT 12/31	

Figure AI-5 Surveillance Report form for recording deficiencies that are conveniently tabulated. Unacceptable results of testing materials with control cultures in a disk susceptibility test are listed. Erratic results with most drugs appeared sporadic, hence no systematic error was suspected. Large zones led to a check of the density of $BaSO_4$ standard. Unacceptably large zones for colistin had been observed during the previous month. Acceptable results were consistently obtained with one of two commercial sources of dehydrated Mueller-Hinton medium (see Figure 6-14, p. 154, for data of 12/03/72).

Use for items when surveillance reveals deficiency.

ITEM Susceptibility Test – Personnel

Deficiency observed: Date 12/15/72

Describe:

Unacceptably small readings obtained with
Gentamicin, Ampicillin, Ceph, Polymyxin
Control data on batch shows no
drugs unacceptable

Date corrective action taken 12/15/72

Nature of corrective action:

Reviewed interpretation of zone
diameters with technologist. Found
that she was selecting target that
fell completely within zone not touching
any portion of growth

Was deficiency corrected? _____ YES ✓ NO Date 12/15/72

If not corrected EXPLAIN

Further surveillance needed (✓)   Reported by JT

Figure AI-6 A report of an erroneous interpretation of control strain zone diameters by a technologist. Current batches of media and disks had been tested previously and found capable of producing proper zone diameters. Zones are read by the placement of a pattern of concentric rings with varying diameters beneath the plate.

SHEET B

Use for items when surveillance reveals deficiency.

ITEM *7/B 4339 Foster 2 door Refrigerator*

Deficiency observed: Date *12/14/72*

Describe:

Alarm Sounded 2 PM Temp 10°C

Date corrective action taken *12/14*

Nature of corrective action:

*Biologicals transferred. Engineering called
freon added biologicals replaced when
temp returned to 8°C. Showed engineer
data noting increases in temp with previous
episodes on monthly cycle. They will check
for leaks*

Was deficiency corrected? ___✓___YES _____NO Date *12/14/72*

If not corrected, EXPLAIN

further Surveillance needed   *AB*

Figure AI-7 Surveillance Report of refrigerator alarm incident; note that proper handling of biologicals was described. Data documented in the surveillance record depicted in Figure 6-9, page 142, was helpful in convincing engineering of the need to search for leaks to prevent future incidents.

222

ITEM	DATE OBSERVED	OBSERVATION	DATE ACTION TAKEN	ACTION TAKEN	RESULTS OF ACTION TAKEN	PROCEDURE CHANGES
ASc	12/6	Control performed but not recorded Antigen lot number not recorded [D]	12/7	Asked tech to show me worksheets daily -This has happened before [D]	Pending	none
ASc	12/22	Did not perform or record control	12/22	Tech said she got it out reviewed it on own sheet but forgot to run it [D]	Will look at day sheets daily again Tech warned about effect on merit appraisal due next month [R]	none

Figure AI-8 A report of the failure to record antigen and control numbers, and later actual control results, from an antistreptolysin titer are tabulated chronologically in this Surveillance Report form. The notation that the problem is "pending" insures that the matter will be reviewed in following month's Surveillance Report. See Figures 6-18 and 6-19, pages 160 and 161, for quality control records from which these errors were derived.

Use for items when surveillance reveals deficiency.

ITEM Typhoid O

Deficiency observed: Date 12/6/72

Describe:

Titer of 40 obtained with Control
Serum — Should have gotten 160

Date corrective action taken 12/6

Nature of corrective action:

Tests repeated with another
control. Correct value obtained —
results reported

Was deficiency corrected? ✓ YES _____ NO Date 12/6/72

If not corrected, EXPLAIN

Figure AI-9 Report of erroneous value obtained for typhoid control serum and corrective action taken (see Figure 6-20, and 6-21, pp. 162, 163).

ITEM	DATE OBSERVED	OBSERVATION	DATE ACTION TAKEN	ACTION TAKEN	RESULTS OF ACTION TAKEN	PROCEDURE CHANGES
Decarboxylase, lysine	12/16	Acid reaction with E.coli. Checked with Media room - forgot to add lysine JF	12/16	New batch made - Personnel reminded to follow procedure carefully JF	new batch 12/16 OK JF	none JF
Decarboxylase lysine	12/21	Exceeded max autoclave time. Was run with 1000 ml vol of Soy broth at same time JF	12/21	pH and control cultures OK So approved media for use. Reminded Media personnel to autoclave different volumes separately JF	don't know - watch future surveillance	none JF
Decarboxylase lysine	12/28	Media Room did not record pH and did not label time temp record. Found out they forgot to check pH. I checked it and found it 5.6 (0.3 low) JF		Rejected batch. Discussed this and other problems with media lately with Supervisor and media room personnel JF	Mary has been out sick and personnel have been working overtime. This may explain rash of errors JF	Temporarily have one technologist work 2 hrs/day in media room until Mary is back JF

Figure AI-10 Surveillance report of errors documented in the worksheet depicted in Figure 6-23, page 165. Note the complete explanation of the observation and action taken.

Use of Lyophilization and Liquid Nitrogen for Storing Cultures

Many inquiries are received regarding equipment and conduct of procedures for storage of cultures either in lyophile or in liquid nitrogen. Workers should learn these procedures by visiting other laboratories where personnel experienced in these techniques can provide instruction and supervised practical experience.

The following material is abstracted from more detailed procedures prepared by Cheryl Rutz, technical supervisor in the author's laboratory. These indicate the equipment that will be required and give sufficient information on procedures to provide the reader with an understanding of the effort, hazards, and special skills needed.

LYOPHILIZATION OF BIOLOGICAL MATERIALS

Principle

The term "lyophile" means solvent loving. This process, termed lyophilization in 1935 by Flosdorf and Mudd, consists of three distinct phases: freezing, sublimation, secondary drying.

Freezing is accomplished by immersing an ampule containing the specimen in a solution (usually ethylene glycol) containing dry ice. The material reaches approximately $-75°C$ and may then be placed on a lyophilizer manifold. Under vacuum, sublimation takes place, transforming the frozen solvent (water) into vapor without passing through the liquid phase. Sublimation occurs when the vapor pressure of a solid becomes greater than the atmospheric pressure and the solid vaporizes. Thus the water is removed from the material being lyophilized and a dry and porous product remains. The heat loss caused by sublimation simultaneously keeps the material frozen until it is dry. Secondary drying refers to the prolonged treatment within the vacuum allowing dehydration to approach completion by removing the final traces of moisture.

Equipment

A. Freeze-dryer (Virtis Company, Inc., Gardiner, N.Y.). This is a stainless steel container with an attached manifold and removable center well (see Figure AII-1). The vacuum in the condenser is maintained by a rubber seal ring which should be lightly greased (Dow Corning, silicone lubricant, high vacuum grease). Tubulations are provided for connection to the secondary condenser and McLeod gauge. The manifold has 24 parts and is connected to the outside wall of the condenser by tubulations. The unit is autoclavable but valves must be removed.

B. Secondary condenser (Virtis Company, Inc.). This is the same as a freeze dryer but slightly smaller and without a manifold. It is also autoclavable.

C. Valves (Virtis Company, Inc.). A faucet-like neoprene valve with a polypropylene stopcock plug, for attaching the ampules to the manifold. These should be decontaminated in a mild disinfectant solution because autoclaving causes neoprene to deteriorate, resulting in loss of vacuum.

D. Hose (Virtis Company, Inc.). A heavy gauge rubber vacuum hose to fit a ¾ in. port is needed.

E. McLeod vacuum gauge (Virtis Company, Inc.). Proper functioning of the pressure gauge is essential. Both the gauge and mercury must be free from dust and the correct amount of mercury must be used. The gauge holds 9 ml of mercury. To clean the mercury:

1. Empty the mercury into a mortar.
2. Add a moderate amount of dextrose.
3. Mix thoroughly with pestel until the mercury appears clean.
4. Add distilled water to float off the dextrose.
5. Remove the excess water from the surface of the mercury with a Pasteur pipette.
6. Mercury may be replaced in the gauge by using a syringe and needle.

To clean the gauge:

1. After removing mercury from the gauge, rinse with hot detergent using suction.

2. Follow this rinse with a distilled water rinse.
3. Flush the gauge with dilute nitric acid, then rinse it with water and acetone to dry it.
4. Mercury may then be replaced and should reach the 0 line when the gauge is held in a vertical position.

F. Vacuum Pump (Precision Scientific Vacuum Pump, Model 75). The oil level should be checked before each operation. Vacuum pump oil (Precision Scientific Co.) should be used. If all connections are well sealed and a vacuum is being maintained, the pump will run smoothly and quietly.

G. Torch, Type 3A Blowpipe (National Welding Equipment Co.) with 228 N. tips.

1. Attach the airline of the torch to the compressed air source.
2. Attach the gasline to the gas source (general lab supply of natural gas or city gas is sufficient).
3. Turn the gas on, ½ turn, and light with a striker, not a match.
4. Slowly work in air until a clean flame is obtained (may require readjusting the gas).

H. Ampules—glass, 2 ml (Bellco Glass Co.).
I. Nutrient agar slants.
J. Dry ice—10 lbs.
K. Vacuum grease (Dow Corning, Midland, Mich.).
L. Ethylene glycol (Fischer Scientific Co.).
M. Sterile milk.
N. Vortex mixer.

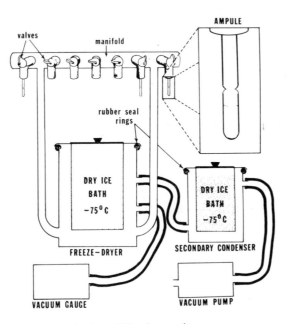

Figure AII-1   Lyphilization equipment.

O. Thermometer (to $-75°C$).

P. Pasteur pipettes (sterile).

Q. Serological pipettes 1 ml (sterile).

R. Biological safety cabinet with air incineration or ultrafiltration.

Connections

Because the drying speed depends on the diffusion rate of the vapor into the condenser, all hose connections should be relatively straight and short. To ensure the best possible vacuum, all hose connections, seal rings, ampules and valve connections should be well greased, using high vacuum grease. The connections should be regreased after every 16 hours of use. After 40 hours of use, all connections should be thoroughly cleaned and regreased.

Procedure

A. On the day prior to lyophilization, cultures should be set up on agar slants and incubated overnight. (Anaerobic cultures are set up in thioglycollate broth and fastidious organisms are planted on chocolate agar slants.) Dry ice must be ordered the day before (10 lbs).

B. Before starting the pump, wipe all moisture off the trap pans and lightly grease all connections with high vacuum grease.

C. Run the pump about 1 hour before beginning lyophilization to create a good vacuum (10 tor or better).

D. Fill the trap pans ⅔ full of ethylene glycol and carefully add small quantities of dry ice to the solution. When the solution approaches $-75°C$, it will become viscous.

E. Pipette 2 ml of sterile milk into the slant tubes and suspend the culture using a loop. Vortex gently.

F. When the vacuum reaches 10 tor, pipette 0.5 ml of the culture suspension into an ampule using a Pasteur pipette.

G. Place the ampule on the Vortex mixer and immediately dip in it dry ice solution for a few seconds while the culture suspension is thrown up on the walls of ampule. Mix and freeze again to form a frozen shell on the inside of the ampule. Repeat this procedure several times until the entire culture is frozen. (Try to keep the culture below the scored area of the ampule.)

H. Place the ampule onto the manifold and slowly open the valve.

I. Do not place another ampule on the machine until the vacuum has again reached 10 tor.

J. When extraction is completed, after about 2 hours, burn off the ampules with the torch at the constricted area.

K. To rehydrate the culture the ampules are broken in a biological safety cabinet. Do not use a chemical fume hood. Cover with an alcohol-soaked gauze to minimize airborne contamination. Using a Pasteur pipette, carefully place 1 ml of soybroth in the vial. After mixing, the reconstituted culture is inoculated into tubes of broth (thioglycollate for anaerobes and blood broth for fastidious organisms) and incubated overnight.

L. Most lyophilized cultures may be stored at room temperature. However, *Hemophilus, Neisseria,* and other fastidious organisms should be kept refrigerated.

REFERENCES

Kabat, Elvin and Manfred, Mayer, *Experimental Immunochemistry,* Charles Thomas, Springfield, Ill., 1961.

Simatos, Denise and Louis Rey, "Freeze-drying of Biologic Materials," *Fed. Proc.,* Vol 24, No. 2, Part III, American Society for Experimental Biology, Washington, D.C.

Society of American Bacteriologists, *Manual of Microbiological Methods*, McGraw-Hill, New York, 1957.

Installation and Operating Instructions, Stokes Machine Company, Philadelphia, Pa., 1958.

Virtis Research Equipment Manual, The Virtis Company, Gardiner, N.Y., 1964.

LIQUID NITROGEN STORAGE

Purpose

Storage of cultures in liquid nitrogen is a rapid method of almost maintenance-free, long term preservation of bacteria and protozoa.

Equipment

A. L-D 30 Liquid nitrogen container (Union Carbide). This is a portable-vacuum insulated container originally designed for the artificial insemination industry (Figure AII-2). Constructed of welded aluminum with a plastic neck tube, the fully loaded unit weighs 90 lbs and can be easily moved about on an accessory roller base. The insulated cap can be locked in place and still permit the venting of vaporized nitrogen. The unit stores about 1500 0.7 ml cryules (Wheaton glass) at $-320°F$ above the liquid level.

The storage canisters are held in place at the bottom of the LD-30 by a "spider" and at the top by numbered slots in an index ring.

B. Cannisters for liquid nitrogen container (10) (Linde Division, Union Carbide Corporation).

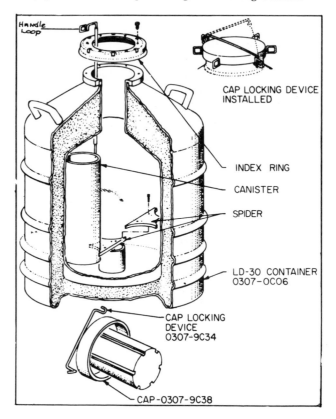

Figure AII-2   LD-30 liquid nitrogen container.

   C. Scored 0.7 ml cryules (Wheaton glass) of special borosilicate glass (each cane holds 6 cryules).

   D. Six place aluminum canes (Shurbend Manufacturing Company) (each canister holds approximately 25 canes).

   E. Glass sealing apparatus.

 1. Welding torch (W-200 Purox Oxy-acetylene torch, Union Carbide), No. 12 welding head.
 2. Oxygen regulator (R-412 O_2 regulator, Presto-lite, Union Carbide).
 3. Oxygen tank (rented, local welding distributor).
 4. A $12\frac{1}{2}$ ft twin hose ($\frac{3}{16}$) (Purox, Union Carbide).
 5. Gas supply (hospital gas supply, propylene and acetylene).
 6. Oxweld No. 33 Spectacle shade AA3 OH (local welding distributor).
 7. Plastic face mask—full face coverage (2).
 8. Long sleeved asbestos gloves (2 pairs) hospital stock or Chieftain.
 9. Autoclave glove, American Hospital Supply Corp.
10. Glove clamps (hospital stock).
11. Scrub gown (hospital stock).
12. Jumpsuit (Angelica).

F. Liquid nitrogen (Linde Division, Union Carbide Corporation) This can be obtained from hospital supply or from a local distributor. Liquid nitrogen has several chemical characteristics. It does not react readily with other elements. It neither burns nor supports combustion. It combines with some of the more active metals, such as calcium, sodium, and magnesium, to form nitrides. Physically, it is colorless, odorless, tasteless, slightly soluble in water, and a poor conductor of heat and electricity. The liquid is colorless, odorless, slightly lighter than water, nonmagnetic, and does not produce toxic or irritating vapors. Its boiling point at 1 Atm = $-320.4°F$. Its volume of expansion, liquid to gas is 696.5 to 1, percentage by volume in air, 78.09%.

Safety Precautions

Contact with Liquid Nitrogen

Always handle liquid nitrogen carefully. At its extremely low temperature it can produce an effect on the skin similar to a burn. When spilled on a surface it tends to cover it completely and intimately and, therefore, cool a large area. The gases issuing from these liquids are also extremely cold and can produce burns. Delicate tissues, such as those of the eyes, can be damaged by exposure to these cold gases that is too brief to affect the skin of the hands or face.

Boiling and splashing always occurs when charging a warm container or when inserting objects into the liquid. Always perform these operations SLOWLY to minimize boiling and splashing.

Whenever liquids are being handled be sure that there is a hose or a large open container of water nearby. Use the water to wash off any area of the body that is accidentally splashed with liquid nitrogen.

Never allow any unprotected part of the body to touch uninsulated pipes or vessels containing liquefied atmospheric gases; the extremely cold metal may stick fast and tear the flesh when attempting to withdraw from it. Use tongs to withdraw objects immersed in liquid nitrogen, and handle the tongs and the object carefully. In addition to the hazard of burns or skin sticking to cold materials, objects that are soft and pliable at room temperatures usually become very hard and brittle at these low temperatures and are very easily broken.

Protective Clothing

Protect the eyes with a face shield or safety goggles (safety spectacles without side shield do *not* give adequate protection). Always wear gloves when handling anything that is, or may have been, in contact with liquid.

Asbestos gloves are recommended, but leather gloves may also be used. The gloves should fit loosely, so that they can be thrown off quickly if liquid should spill or splash into them. When handling liquids in open containers, it is advisable to wear high-top shoes. Trousers (which should be cuffless if possible) should be worn *outside* the shoes. Long sleeves are essential.

Ventilation in Work and Storage Areas

Store and use liquid nitrogen only in a well-ventilated place. If enough nitrogen gas evaporates from the liquid in an unventilated space, the percentage of oxygen in the air may become dangerously low. *When the oxygen concentration in the air is sufficiently low, a man can become unconscious without sensing any warning symptoms, such as dizziness.* If he remains in this atmosphere long enough, death can result.

Keep in mind that nitrogen buildup is most likely to occur when the room is closed, for example, overnight. If there is any doubt about the amount of oxygen in a room, ventilate the room completely before entering it. Never dispose of waste nitrogen in a confined area or a place that someone else may enter.

Solution of Oxygen in Liquid Nitrogen:

Liquid nitrogen is colder than liquid oxygen. Therefore, if it is exposed to the air, oxygen from the air may condense in the liquid nitrogen. If this continues for any length of time, the oxygen dissolved in the liquid will create a combustibility hazard. Most liquid nitrogen containers are entirely closed except for a small neck area, and the nitrogen gas issuing from the surface of the liquid forms a barrier that keeps air away from the liquid and prevents oxygen contamination.

Using a Torch

Attach the welding head to the torch. Next, attach the oxygen hose to the torch and the regulator. Then attach the acetylene hose to the gas supply and the torch.

After proper operating pressure has been established on the oxygen regulator, open the torch oxygen valve one quarter of a turn. Open the torch acetylene one full turn. Using a friction lighter, light the gas at the tip. Do NOT use a match. Slowly open the torch oxygen valve. Throttle the acetylene valve to obtain a blue flame without a trace of yellow.

If acetylene is used, the flame temperature will be approximately 6000°F.

If propane or city gas mixtures are used, the temperature will be approximately 4500–5000°F.

To shut off the torch, close the torch *acetylene* valve, then the torch oxygen valve.

Operating Precautions

Backfire

The flame may go out with a loud pop; this is called a "backfire." The flames of the W-200 are resistant to the occasional backfires normally caused by the use of a very short flame, or by overheating of the head or nozzle. Other common causes of backfires are: (*a*) operating the torch at insufficient gas pressure; (*b*) touching the work with the tip of the welding head or the nozzle; (*c*) a loose welding head connection or a loose nozzle; and (*d*) dirt on the head seat or on the nozzle seat.

Flashback

When the flame burns back inside the torch or cutting attachment, usually with a shrill hissing or squealing sound, it is called a "flashback." The advanced design of the W-200 makes flashbacks almost impossible. However, if a flashback should occur, proceed as follows:

1.   Immediately close the torch oxygen valve.
2.   Close the torch acetylene valve.
3.   After a moment, relight the torch in the usual manner.

Working Set-up

It is neither practical nor safe to hold the torch in one hand and the cryule in the other to seal because of the size of the cryule, the heat of the flame, and the inconvenience of setting the torch down safely while it is in operation. A simple apparatus can easily be set up for securely holding the torch safely, using a support stand and a utility camp.

Caution: The torch should not be aimed at anything flammable in the near vicinity since the ignition flame can be large if the operator is careless. A fireproof heat shield is recommended.

Procedure

Preparation of the Specimen

Cryules should be sterilized. Colonies can be picked from any young culture (12–18 hours) and suspended in a nutrient medium. A broth suspension can be easily inserted in the cryule using a sterile Pasteur pipette or with a syringe and needle (1½ in.). The advantage of the needle and syringe is facility in measuring the volume inserted; using the thin needle also avoids contamination of neck glass. Take care not to contaminate the glass surface of the neck with foreign material (media, cotton, etc.) as this interferes with sealing the ampule.

Sealing the Ampule

If the torch has been suspended in a stationary position, hold the ampule in hand and rotate evenly and moderately fast for almost a complete turn. It is essential to wear protective glasses (they need not be very dark) to reduce the glare of the sodium flame. The sealing process takes a few seconds.

The ampule should not be held in the flame after it appears melted and sealed since the expanding air (due to the high heat intensity of the torch) causes the soft glass to pop, leaving a small air vent that is not easily patched. It is advisable to start again with a new ampule if this happens. If the culture sample is small, let the ampule cool, open it, and transfer the contents to a new ampule.

The seal should be inspected under a dissecting microscope. If this is not readily available, a reverse 10 × 15 ocular may be used. The ampule should be rotated in an indirect light source for this inspection.

High intensity heat must be used for sealing because the ampule should be melted closed as quickly as possible. If cooler slower methods are used, the hot air inside the ampule and the glass itself will heat, not only causing damage to the culture and the operator's hands, but also leaving a gaping hole through which the hot air in the ampule will escape. If ampules are not completely sealed, nitrogen will flow into the ampule in storage. When this ampule is removed from liquid nitrogen, the liquid will rapidly boil to gas and cause an "explosion" of the ampule when the gas attempts to expand. Precautions for the "explosion" are described in the section concerning the removal of the ampule.

Labeling and Identification of Ampules and Canes

Ampules are labeled with adhesive tape and an indelible pen. The adhesive tape is placed on the upper taper of the ampule neck because this does not interfere with the prongs of the cane which grip the ampule in storage. The canes are made of aluminum and can be easily labeled with a punch or an engraving tool.

Insertion of Cryules and Canes in Liquid Nitrogen

Cryules are placed on the cane. The operator should wear a face mask and gloves for the next operation. The cane is placed in the canister. To remove a canister, lift the handle loop out of its slot and tilt the canister into the neck tube opening. To replace the canister, tilt it in the direction of the handle slot so that the canister bottom slips into the recess in the spider beneath that slot. Avoid unnecessary loss of refrigeration by not completely removing the canister from the necktube.

Precautions Prior to Removal of Cryule

A stainless steel container with a loose, but attached top should be positioned level with the top of the refrigerator necktube opening. It should be filled halfway with disinfectant solution. The container and disinfectant provide a place to put the cryule as it is removed from the cane. The fluid cushions the fall of the cryule. If the cryule explodes, the container confines the explosion. The disinfectant reduces the hazard of contamination if the container is left undisturbed for 30–60 minutes after an explosion.

Removing a Cryule from Liquid Nitrogen

Lift the handle loop and tilt the canister into the necktube opening, raise the canister, and select a cane. Remove the cane and place it, cryule down, over the open canister. Hold the bottom of the cane with the free glove to steady it over the canister containing the disinfectant. Place a towel clamp around the cane, but behind the cryule neck (do not allow the clamp to lock), and pull toward the base of the cryule. This partially displaces the cryule from its position on the cane. Remove the towel clamp from the cane, and gently push the cryule into the disinfectant by pushing the clamp through the oval opening on the back of the cane. Put the lid on the disinfectant container. Replace the cane and canister.

Removing a Culture from a Cryule

Let the cryule thaw in the covered disinfectant container for 5 minutes. Remove the cryule and wrap it, right side up, in a 2 × 2 in. gauze pad.

Break at the stricture, unwrap, and throw away the top in the disinfectant. Remove the culture from the Pasteur pipette or syringe and needle. Transfer it to a culture medium.

Care and Maintenance

The level of liquid in the container can be measured with a wooden yard-stick inserted to the top of the spider. Withdraw after 5–10 seconds and note the length of the frosted section, then refer to a conversion table to determine the volume of the remaining liquid nitrogen. The temperature in the supernatant vapor phase is about −270°F. Any liquid that is left in the tank, is at this temperature. Usually no distinction is made between storage in the liquid or vapor phase.

Never use hollow rods or tubes as dip sticks for measuring liquid level. When a warm tube is inserted into liquid nitrogen, liquid spouts from the top of the tube because of the rapid expansion of the liquid inside the tube.

Determining Liquid Contents

Container Liquid Level (in above Spider)	Volume in Liters of Liquid Nitrogen
0	2.7 or less
1	5.1
2	7.5
3	9.8
4	12.2
5	14.6
6	17.0
7	19.4
8	21.8
9	24.2
10	26.6
11	29.0
12	31.1
13	31.8

REFERENCES

Instructions for Ld-30 Liquid Nitrogen Container, Form 13-655-A, Linde Division, Union Carbide Corporation, Speedway, Ind.

Liquified atmosphere gases, precautions and safe practices, ibid

Instructions for Purox W-200 Welding Torch, Form 9773-G, ibid

Marymont, J. H. and J. P. Smith, "Topics in Microbiology: The use of liquid nitrogen," *Am J. Clin. Path.*, Vol. 51, 676–677 (1969).

Smith, John P., personal communication, Wesley Medical Center, Wichita, Kans.

BIBLIOGRAPHY

Chapter 1

No references.

Chapter 2

1. W. G. Johanson, A. K. Pierce, and J. P. Sanford, "Changing Pharyngeal bacterial flora of hospitalized patients," *N. Engl. J. Med.*, 281:1137–1140, 1969.

2. M. R. Moody, V. M. Young, G. D. Vermuelen, and J. W. Gerster, "The presence of *Enterobacter* and *Klebsiella sp.* in cancer patients and their subsequent role as pathogens," *Abstr. Ann. Meet. Am. Soc. Microbiol*, 1973.

3. R. B., Lindberg, A. D. Mason, Jr., and B. A. Pruitt, Jr., "*Providencia stuartii* as a major factor in burn unit infections," *Abstr. Ann. Mett. Am. Soc. Microbiol.*, 1973.

4. D. S. deJohngh, J. W. Loftis, G. S. Green, J. A. Shively, and T. M. Minckler, *Am. J. Clin. Pathol.*, 49:424–428, 1968.

5. F. Deland and H. N. Wagner, Jr., "Automated radiometric detection of bacterial growth in blood cultures," *J. Lab. Clin. Med.*, 74:529, 1970.

6. New blood culture techniques, "Septicemia: Laboratory and Clinical Aspects," A. Balows, Ed. American Lecture Series in Clinical Microbiology, Charles C. Thomas, Springfield, Ill., 1973.

7. A. S. Werner, C. G. Cobbs, D. Kaye, and E. W. Hook, "Studies on the bacteremia of bacterial endocarditis," *JAMA*, 202:127, 1967.

8. H. D. Hochstein, W. R. Kirkam, and V. M. Young, "Recovery of more than one organism in septicemias," *N. Engl. J. Med.*, 273:488, 1965.

9. W. G. Johanson, A. K. Pierce, and J. P. Sanford, "Changing Pharyngeal flora of hospitalized patients," *N. Engl. J. Med.*, 281:1137, 1969.

10. E. Barrett-Connor, "The non value of sputum culture in the diagnosis of pneumococcal pneumonia," *Am. Rev. Respir. Dis.*, 103:845–848, 1971.

11. R. C. Bartlett and A. Melnick, "Usefulness of Gram stain and routine and quantitative

culture of sputum in patients with and without acute respiratory infection," *Conn. Med.*, 34:347–351, 1970.

12. F. A. Loda, W. A. Clyde, Jr., W. P. Glezen, R. J. Senior, C. I. Sheaffer, and F. W. Denny, Jr., "Studies on the role of viruses, bacteria and M. pneumoniae as causes of lower respiratory tract infections in children," *J. Pediatr.*, 72:161–176, 1968.

13. J. Scanlon. "The early detection of neonatal sepsis by examination of liquid obtained from the external ear canal," *J. Pediatr.*, 79:247–249, 1971.

14. A. Ramos, and L. Stern, "Relationship of premature rupture of the membranes to gastric fluid aspitate in the newborn," *Am. J. Obstetri. Gynecol.*, 105:1247–1251, 1969.

15. D. E. Polter, J. D. Boyle, L. Miller, and S. M. Finegold, "Anaerobic bacteria as cause of the blind loop syndrome: a case report with observations, on response to antibacterial agents," *Gastroenterology*, 54:1148–1154, 1968.

16. J. C. Colbeck, "Control of infections in hospitals," American Hospital Association, Chicago, 1962.

17. G. F. Grady and G. T. Keusch, "Pathogenesis of bacterial diarrheas," *N. Engl. J. Med.*, 285:831–841, 891–900, 1971.

18. E. H. Kass, "Asymptomatic infections of the urinary tract," *Trans. Assoc. Am. Physicians*, 69:56, 1956.

19. D. Wachtel, W. Witzleb, and H. Thieler, "The importance of suprapubic bladder aspiration in bacteriologic organisms," *Wein. Klin. Wschr.*, 84:344–347, 1972.

20. T. S. Stamey, D. E. Gavan, and J. M. Palmer, "The localization and treatment of urinary tract infections: the role of Bacteroidal urine levels as opposed to serum levels," *Medicine*, 44:1–36, 1965.

21. W. A. Craig and C. M. Kunin, "Quantitative urine culture method using a plastic "paddle" containing dual media," *Appl. Microbiol.*, 23:919–922, 1972.

22. E. M. Mackay-Scollay, "A simple quantitative and qualitative microbiological screening test for bacteriuria," *J. Clin. Pathol.*, 22:651–653, 1969.

23. C. R. Amies and A. Corpas, "A preservative for urine specimens in transit to the Bacteriological laboratory," *J. Med. Microbiol.*, 4:362–365, 1971.

24. J. T. Headington and B. Beyerlein, "Anaerobic bacteria in routine urine culture," *J. Clin. Pathol.*, 19:573–576, 1966.

25. J. W. Segura, P. P. Kelalis, W. J. Martin, and L. H. Smith, "Anaerobic bacteria in the urinary tract," *Mayo Clin. Proc.*, 47:30–33, 1972.

26. J. A. Guilbeau, Jr. and I. G. Schaub, "Uterine culture technique," *Am. J. Obstetri. Gynecol.*, 58:407–410, 1949.

27. R. C. Bartlett, "Control of Hospital Associated Infections," *Progress in Clinical Pathology*, M. Stefanini, Ed., Grune & Stratton, New York, 1972.

Chapter 3

No references.

Chapter 4

1. J. Petralli, E. Russell, A. Kataoka, and T. Merigan, "On-line computer quality control of antibiotic-sensitivity testing," *N. Engl. J. Med.*, 283:735–738, 1970.

2. T. L. Gaven and C. A. Ma, "Computer assisted identification of Enterobacteriaceae," *Abstr. Ann. Meet. Am. Soc. Microbiol.*, 1972.

Chapter 5

1. "Health Service Occupations: Occupational needs: educational requirements" Division of Vocational Education, State Department of Education, Labor Education Center, The University of Connecticut, 1967.
2. Arthur E. Rappaport, "Manual for laboratory planning and design," The College of American Pathologists, Chicago, 1960.
3. R. C. Bartlett, G. O. Carrington, and C. Mielert, "Quality Control in Clinical Microbiology—Revised," Commission on Continuing Education, American Society of Clinical Pathologists, Chicago, 1970.
4. "A workload recording method for clinical laboratories," College of American Pathologists, Chicago, 1970.

Chapter 6

1. Federal Register 33 F.R. 15297–15303, November 15, 1968.
2. Joanne Packer, Ruth C. Russell, R. P. Henke, and E. R. Jennings, "Stability of prepared microbiological culture media," *Abstr. Ann. Meet. Am. Soc. Microbio.*, 1972.
3. A. W. Bauer, W. M. Kirby, J. C. Sherris, and M. Turck, "Antibiotic susceptibility testing by a standardized single disk method," *Am. J. Clin. Pathol.* 45:493–496, 1966.
4. A. L. Barry, F. Gracia, and L. D. Thrupp, "An improved single disk method for testing the antibiotic susceptibility of rapidly growing pathogens," *Am. J. Clin. Pathol.*, 53:149–158, 1970.
5. R. C. Bartlett and Mary Mazens, "Analytical variability in the single disk antimicrobial susceptibility test," *Am. J. Clin. Pathol.* 59:376–383, 1973.
6. R. C. Bartlett and Mary Mazens, "Effect of Plate Size and location of disk on zone diameter in the disc antimicrobial susceptibility test," *Appl. Microbiol.*, 22:372–376, 1971.
7. "Performance standards for antimicrobial disk susceptibility tests, as used in clinical laboratories," National committee for Clinical Laboratory Standards, Los Angeles, 1972.

Index

Numbers in italics refer to illustrations.

245